Dr. Gene Dagnone is professor emeritus of Emergency Medicine at Queen's University in Kingston, Canada. He has authored and co-authored a wide range of emergency medicine articles in the medical and health services journals in Canada, United States and Great Britain. He has served on the editorial board of two emergency medicine journals. His learning, teaching, research and clinical care experience spans half a century.

In clinical practice, teaching and research, Dr. Dagnone and his emergency department colleagues are in search of the 'best answer'. When answers are not available or weak, in terms of sensitivity and specificity, there are always better questions to ask and other possibilities to consider. The sharing of this anthology of experiences 'in listening in the emergency department' focuses on the trust and translation of the listening that occurs between caregiver and patient, caregiver and 'next of kin', caregiver with each other.

Dedication

This anthology, "A Call To Listen – The Emergency Department Visit" is dedicated to Goe, our father, our first teacher, a devoted caregiver and an ardent storyteller.

Acknowledgements:

Dr. Jacqueline Duffin, Hannah Chair, History of Medicine at Queen's University, Kingston Canada. Your enthusiasm and direction was pivotal in encouraging me to get these stories told.

Laura Scott, Queen's University Bracken Library for help in the medical literature search.

Chelsea Humphries for excellent assistance in copyediting.

The many physician and nurse colleagues in Emergency Medicine – thank you for sharing your talents and your commitment to making a difference in so many lives each day!

The clinical and academic mentors who patiently guided my path in seeking out the vital histories of my patients.

Joel, Damon, Vico and Marla – may your own stories as caregivers bring joy to each chapter of your lives.

Danielle – Your love and encouragement make all things possible.

Dr. Gene Dagnone

A Call to Listen –
The Emergency
Department Visit

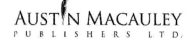

A CIP catalogue record for this title is available from the British Library.

ISBN 9781786293862 (Paperback)
ISBN 9781786293879 (Hardback)
ISBN 9781786293886 (E-Book)
www.austinmacauley.com

First Published (2017)
Austin Macauley Publishers Ltd.
25 Canada Square
Canary Wharf
London
E14 5LQ

Contents

Prologue

A storyteller's last words continue to resonate with his son.

Introduction

The members of the emergency department team and the patient's 'next of kin' are brought together to listen to the patient's story.

Anthology of Vital Histories

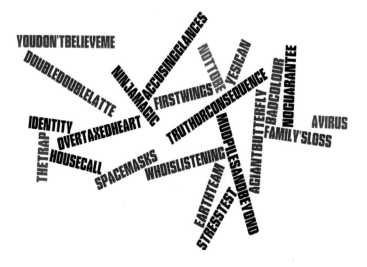

Last Words: Prologue

"Dr. Peter, are you finished handover? There's a long distance call that the hospital operator thinks you should take. Extension 359."

"Thanks, Edna. I'll take it at the desk."

I pick up the phone.

"This is the Regina Pasqua Hospital calling. We are looking for any relative of a Goe ...I will spell his last name: S-U-B-I-T-O. Do you know how we can contact his family?"

I take the call. It's about my father. The emergency department nurse assures me that she just received handover from the day team and my father is in stable condition. He is being admitted for a heart condition. I can't speak to him until he gets to his assigned bed. He had some shortness of breath overnight; no pain, nothing serious. She says "he'll be in the coronary care unit for a few days". She asks for any past history and family history I wish to add. She will let Dad know that we talked. She records my cell number. She seems to be in a hurry. I express thanks for the call. Why am I filled with dread and doubt?

What does the ECG⊕ show?

I call back. The ECG shows no acute changes. It is considered to be normal except for a left bundle branch block⊕.

I tell the emergency department charge nurse that the 'Bundle Branch Block' is a new finding. It was not there when he had his last overall check-up at his family doctor six months ago.

A few days become a week. Every day, the message seems to be "not yet; your father is not ready to go home". I book the two flights to check for myself.

A typical prairie, first of November snowstorm greets my evening arrival. On the final approach, the city lights cast an array of halos in a much too early collage of Christmas cards. The terminal screens indicate that all further flights in and out are cancelled.

The taxi driver asks where I'm coming from and what I do. He is taken back with my requested destination. Yes, I am a doctor going to a hospital from an airport, but I am coming to visit family.

Each street sign, framed by the frosted taxi windowpanes, brings back a cascade of vivid memories from long ago. Each intersection augurs a new and different array of pleasant remembrances for this community's once west side youth. These recollections of friends, family and places have survived the ensuing five

---

⊕ **ECG** – electrocardiogram
⊕ **Bundle Branch Block** – appearance on the electrocardiogram that identifies the location of a defect in the conduction system of the heart

decades. The baffles of my mind try to complete the lyrics to 'Four Strong Winds', a pleading prairie melody of the mid-1960s. The singer longs to hope that permanent separation will not occur, but it is apparent that little optimism remains. You are drawn to repeat the melody over again, to see if, possibly, there has been a change of heart.

I reach the hospital's coronary care unit during their 10 p.m. handover. I introduce myself and accept an invitation to hear the nursing staff update for my father.

"Mr. Subito, Goe, as he likes to be called, was admitted seven days ago due to overnight shortness of breath. His cardiogram shows no serious changes from earlier ECGs but manifests a Left Bundle Branch that was not previously evident. He has some x-ray evidence of left ventricular heart failure, which has improved with diuretics⊕. The rise in his cardiac enzyme markers did not peak until yesterday indicating some continuing heart muscle injury. Also, his discharge has been delayed because his kidney function has been declining. Hopefully that will stabilize now that his diuretics have been reduced. He denies any pain and was able to sleep with two pillows last night. His vital signs and his monitored heart rhythm remain stable. Yesterday's measurement of the ejection fraction⊕ is reasonable at forty per cent. He repeatedly asks about his blood pressure reading. If anything, it has been running on the low side. 'Good Italian food,' he is quick to explain. He is alert, pays attention to every detail and likes to tease. He has started to tell stories."

⊕ **Diuretic** – medication that increases fluid loss through its action on the kidneys

Visiting hours are flexible. Dad seems fine for his eighty-three years, sitting up in bed, not short of breath, perhaps a few pounds less than last year. He keeps repeating, "I am ready to go home".

Dad and I spend the next hour catching up on his grandchildren's achievements, confirming his apparent lack of cardiac symptoms, and reassuring each other. He asks for the hundredth time: "When will you move back home and start a practice? When do you plan to retire?" He knows the answers. He has heard them before.

"Probably never. I'm not interested in moving, changing or retiring. I love my work as an emergency physician even after more than forty years." I explain how my practice, teaching and research in emergency medicine reward me immensely. I boast, "Today, many of the brightest medical and nursing students are choosing a career in Emergency Medicine". If history could be rewritten for him, I say that he would relish being on our emergency department team dealing with the endless array of diagnostic challenges, and management decisions that we face each hour of each day. "There are always surprises, and sad stories sometimes, but mostly uplifting tales."

As I prepare to take my leave for the evening, Dad admonishes me for having my cell phone on.

I respond quickly: "It doesn't affect cardiac monitors; I wear it at the hospital all the time." I also explain that the cell phone gives me confidence that my children—his grandchildren—can always contact me. I mention that he was lucky that he did not have to deal with sudden emergencies when his children were growing up.
Dad pauses; he smirks, and cannot let it go.

"You know son ... what you do not know about life emergencies would fill a book. You forget. We had to take care of our own emergencies. We didn't have the luxury of hospitals, ambulances, or fancy doctors."

This is Dad's entry. This is an open invitation. I should not have gone here. He loves telling stories... stories of ghosts... 'stregas', near death scenarios, holy water revivals. Which one will he pick to begin? He has lived through them all: war scenarios, desperate hunger, natural disasters, infectious disease, and life threatening traumas.

Almost always told in his native tongue, his audience is anyone that might listen. His grandchildren have learned to feign language incomprehension. Each story has a solution. My brother, sister and I collectively recall that the solutions are most often generated through a distraction caused by a trustworthy donkey, prayers to the Madonna or pleadings to St. Anthony for lost things and lost causes.

He begins. Of course, it's the beggar woman—with the crying baby... hiding under the late evening shadows of the bridge—as German soldiers pillage everything in their path. The crying child will give away the hiding place. The crying must stop. Mother has no further milk to give the hungry child. Death is imminent. Surely someone somewhere would think to portray this tragic futile situation and the unexpected solution in a movie.

I wait for evidence of the approaching punch line, recalling the near completion of the tale. I push my chair back; I resist. I roll my eyes. I look down. I look up. I count the ceiling tiles.

"Yes, Dad, I hear you, but I had better go now. The nurse at the desk is sending me a message that she wants you to get some sleep."

Dad switches to his slow Italian dialect with what can only be translated: "As always, you guys have too much book learning…it swells your head so much, your ears don't know how to listen."

"Thanks once again for the compliment, Dad. You've mentioned it before."

"Have you ever listened?" he asks.

"Yes, Dad, I hear you. I will be back early tomorrow morning. I have arranged to talk to your heart doctor when she comes on her rounds. Have some rest now. You are looking good; I think you may be able to go home soon. Let me grab a few winks myself—just worked a stretch of late evenings. I will be here for a few days. Perhaps I can now share some of my own stories with you. Bet I can stump you on a few of them. You will have to help me translate some of the medical terms into Italian. We have lots of time."

My clinical mind is telling me that Dad is fine; he is back to his old self. His monitored vital signs are within normal range. He doesn't need to take up a Coronary Care Unit bed. He can tell his stories at home.

My dad's last words to me were, "Your ears don't know how to listen; have you ever listened?"

We Are Called to Listen:

Introduction

"This is General Hospital Emergency Department calling. We are looking for any relative of a David Stone. Are you related to him? Do you know how we can contact his family?"

A most unwelcomed intrusion to our day. Fear floods through every vein. Doubt and anger quickly follow. Relax! Someone may be playing a joke on you. Do I recognize the voice? How do I begin to answer?

Who is David Stone? A son? A father? A brother? When was the last time that I saw him?

Personal visits to community emergency departments continually reinforce the notion that strange frenetic activity occurs within those walled caverns. Media portrayals of trauma and arrested life scenarios serve as constant reminders that I never want to receive a call from there, let alone go there.

These words, "We are looking for…" are crackling across our stratosphere every minute of every hour from emergency departments, both near and far. Will the next ring from my phone deliver the words that summon me to the emergency department? On receiving such a call, the reflex reaction is disbelief followed by silence. Do I accept this question without doubting, without concern, without screaming? I did not ask to play this game of tag. Silence gives way to a stuttered response.

Can I prepare myself for that inevitable emergency department call or visit? Can I just accept that what will be, will be? Can I forgive myself for not wanting to go there, or to be in that place?

Caregivers in the emergency department and the summoned recipients of the call abruptly enter into an indispensable relationship. Almost always strangers to each other, they are now required to listen to private and personal information that they, reluctantly but most assuredly, need to share with each other. In the emergency department setting, whether we are a patient, a doctor, a nurse, a parent, a teacher, a student or a distant 'next of kin', nothing can be learned without listening. We must dare to ask. Listening will require our ears to hear and our eyes to see. Moreover, the translation of what we are hearing, seeing and remembering needs to be unconditionally shared with these strangers. The time for this sharing is not unlimited. Are we up to the task of 'listening to each other'?

Emergency department nurses and doctors are expected to be proficient in listening. Listening is the constant within the equation of their decision-making. The 'next of kin', and those assisting, are able to provide clues and introduce new considerations that were not immediately evident on the caregiver's first encounter with the patient. This further information could alter the approach to investigations and interventions. What facts are missing? What actions avoid further harm? How is the information interpreted? What are mere background noises? How are distractions ignored? What assurance can we offer to the patient and family members? Can the caregiver learn from other caregivers sharing past experiences of poor and good listening?

Much that emergency caregivers hear is private and should remain so. A family member's fears differ from a caregiver's concerns. Reaching back in time, our profession as emergency care providers, much like our personal life, is constantly challenged by the words each of us has heard more than once. With each new patient encounter, I am aware of the echo of my father's allegation: "You don't know how to listen!"

There is no body of medical literature that specifically addresses the importance of an emergency department caregiver and the 'next of kin' listening to each other when a health emergency is first recognized. Emergency medicine journals present individual cases and multi-case reviews noting that a significant root cause of litigation in the emergency department setting is attributable to items in the history that are ignored, not available or misinterpreted. ([1234]) In the preface to Rosen's Textbook of Emergency Medicine, 8th edition ([5]), the emergency department caregiver is advised, *"Every medical encounter must be individualized, and every patient must be approached on a case-by-case basis"*. Publications ([67]) from Continuous Quality Improvement initiatives are beginning to recognize the benefits of the reciprocal listening that occurs between the care providers and the 'next of kin' in the emergency department. The 'CanMeds

---

1- 7 Medical Literature References

Physician Competency Framework' describes the knowledge, skills and abilities that physicians are expected to deploy. In the emergency department setting, the 'Communicator' and the 'Collaborator' roles are paramount for each caregiver.

Each emergency care worker has heard a multitude of 'tales from the crypts' from their colleagues. With each telling, some extra fact or twist is added. The stories are meant mainly to scare the novices in the field, sometimes to encourage caution. Most often, however, they declare how ingenious a caregiver can be in spite of the hopelessness of the presented situation. When published, the titles are likely to include provocative words such as: real, true, blood, miracles, mayhem, angels, inspiring, and amazing. As caregivers, as teachers and as learners, each member of each emergency department team will vividly recall similar presentations that they have encountered. These snapshots in time give us opportunities for learning more about the lives of our patients and the subtle nuances built into the practice of our chosen medical specialty. Many of these same scenarios have informed specialty examination questions for our emergency medicine residents and nurses. With each reading, new questions arise. Each passage reveals one or more questions that draw attention to the shared listening lessons that are exemplified in the particular emergency department visit. A list of Selected Readings for Emergency Department Listeners[⊕⊕] is appended.

The emergency department team operates best with a quick presumptive diagnosis and practiced protocols. The translation of unexpected pieces of information needs to be completed expeditiously. For each team member, there

---

[⊕ ⊕] Selected Readings for Emergency Department Listeners

is always another question, a better question. Definitive answers may have to wait. At some point during the emergency department visit, the caregiver and the 'next of kin' ask for input, seek clarification, and request confirmation from each other. Who can judge how well they listen to each other? Will the caregiver and the 'next of kin' come to the same translation of the listening they have shared with each other?

While emergency department nurses and physicians understand the fears and misgivings of family members, they are obliged to remain focussed on what needs to be done. What further information can be gleaned; what action is immediately required. The listening must produce facts that can be acted upon. The listening must help steer the course of positive action.

Our fathers and mothers always emphasized listening when they, as our first teachers, tutored us. That worked well. They let us listen to everything that was important and they taught us how to measure what was important. Then they let us go to school, and more school, and we learned to listen to even more special things that had an increasingly high measure of importance. Whether care providers or 'next of kin', we are faced with the decision of having to select what is important to listen to or ask at any given moment.

The memory bank of this storyteller's son spans a half-century of learning and teaching alongside valued colleagues and learners in emergency medicine. The selected tales are a small sample of the recurring encounters that repeat themselves on a minute-to-minute basis each hour of each day in each emergency department. This anthology is presented as the recollections of brief communications at a fixed time in the workings of a busy emergency department. The stories provide examples of the value of good listening and the consequences of either not listening, or hurried and faulty translations. There is a final common checkpoint for the receiver, the caller, the caregiver, the patient, and the 'next of kin'. "How well do you listen?" This assortment of actual emergency department interactions attempts to capture that aspirant moment when both the family member and the emergency care provider seek space, time, understanding, empathy, good listening and accurate translation.

The dates, details, names, roles (of individual patients, family members and team care providers) and the sequence of the presentations are altered in each scenario to protect the identity of the patients and their families.

The chaotic din within the crowded corridors and canopied spaces silences many voices that need to be heard. All too often, the emergency department entrance door or the initial phone call to the 'next of kin' momentarily triggers the mute button of their knowledge about the patient and past relevant events.

The recipient of the call to the emergency department faces a flotilla of inner voices as he or she listens to the caller and approaches the threshold of the emergency department:
- "Let it not be…"
- "I should have…"
- "I should not have…"

Each story presents the same cast of characters: the patient with a chief complaint, the 'next of kin' (James, Mr. or Mrs. James) and the members of the emergency care team:

- Dr. Peter, Dr. Louise, Dr. John
- Nurse Edna or Nurse Edward
- Other team members

Each patient in the emergency department is given an address: a street address ('section A, B, C, or D') and a 'stretcher address ('1, 2, 3').

Throughout this anthology, the patient is accompanied by or requires a call from the emergency department to a responsible 'next of kin'. Ages, speech competencies, physical and emotional needs vary with each individual patient. The caregivers will base the initial management and investigation decisions on the chief complaint, history of the present illness and vital signs. From arrival to discharge, the foundation for making the best clinical decision rests on how well the caregivers utilize listening beyond the hearing and recording of the chief complaint. As emergency nurses and physicians, we are taught to diligently interpret the patient's vital signs (pulse, blood pressure, respiratory rate, general appearance, coma scale, and oxygen saturation). What scale will we use to interpret the vital history? The vital history is always there but it does not reveal itself in gradations of an accepted or recognized scale. The vital history is delivered in words over time by patient, family and caregivers. As each set of words comes forth, new interpretations become possible. A fundamental question needs to be answered: "What caused the patient to come to or be brought to the emergency department?" At the end of each story, the caregivers and the next of kin are left with a second question: "Could 'good listening' have avoided the agony of this visit to or the call from the emergency department?"

In the situations offered in this collection, the 'next of kin' becomes the point person who has been called or directed to the emergency department. James (Mr. or Mrs.) represents the role of the 'next of kin' of a young child, or teenager or an adult. Too often, but not unsurprisingly, s/he is the most uncomfortable character in the encounter. Each scenario gives credence to the submerged anguish that the family member keeps pent inside. From the moment of arrival to final discharge, the 'next of kin' recognizes that the purpose of the visit is under the scrutiny of strangers. The responsibility for what will happen now passes to others. These strangers are the emergency care providers.

Edna or Edward is the emergency department nurse. In the emergency department, Edna or Edward is the first trained professional who reads the play and determines the timing and call for the handoff. S/he is the individual that first determines what needs to be ascertained, in what order, and who needs to know what in what order. Each emergency department nurse works towards the same common goal. S/he is the master, the boss, the referee, and the lines keeper of the emergency department. Every emergency department doctor knows that the play cannot move forward without Edna/Edward's specific call to attention.

For each interaction there is a minimum of two physicians listening, deciding and learning together. Louise is a staff emergency physician who has ten years of experience after five years of residency training. Peter is a staff emergency physician with twelve years of experience after five years' residency. John is a second year emergency medicine resident. He is the bridge between the two staff physicians and the emergency department nurse. John is expected to handle most of the initial interactions with the patient and their family members.

Other members of the team have specifically assigned support roles. The EMS Paramedic has picked up the pieces of a rapidly declining life or seriously injured body and stabilized the essential life parameters. The Ward Clerk is the communications manager, the intersection controller for the team. Both internal and external to the department there is a host of support staff: Respiratory Therapist, Laboratory and X-ray Technicians, and the Security Guard. The Volunteer offers extra physical hands to the emergency department team and shepherds the lost family members into their unrequested spectator role. Cleaners keep us protected from falls and the plague of infection. Pharmacists fill and double check the prescriptions provided to the patients. Consultants and special teams, on site or at regional sites, await mobilization.

'Handover', in the practice of medicine, occurs across all disciplines and specialties. In emergency medicine, handover is a variable combination of the individual and team's verbal summaries, written notes and electronic fact reviews for each patient in the department. Most often handover starts at the main control desk nearest to the electronic and/or paper chart with white board, and computer terminal within reach. When required, the discussion and the new introductions shift to the bedside. Handover in the emergency department provides the plan that communicates the next steps anticipated in a patient's care (admission, discharge, investigation modality, consultation, transfer, follow up arrangements, return instructions). The verbal component varies in terms of the breadth and depth of detail that is provided by the handing over physician and nurse. It is in these moments that the patient situation is characterized by one team member to the others. The focus is on the patient, or the victim, in bed location A3 or D4. The background comments provide a reminder of the physical and personnel constraints under which the emergency department team operates at that moment.

During these summaries, the handover physician and nurse paint the picture for the on-coming members of the team. In this exchange, new insights that eluded the initial assessment can be weighed. Also, during these moments, the missing parts of the vital history come to light more fully and contribute to the story that is unfolding. The equation may need to be adjusted to include the added expressions of the other caregivers in the team. This is also the time that late-arriving family members' input is added to the measure. Support for the plan of investigation and management is affirmed or the new historical details and translations will suggest that new directions need to be considered.

Emergency department care providers are trained to determine what makes sense instead of dwelling on what does not make sense. Their training is geared both to listen and to anticipate, and to do so in the most time effective manner possible. Sharing our most puzzling scenarios also helps us build a better framework to identify and recognize the common recurring obstacles to listening in the emergency department. Each colleague in emergency medicine and emergency nursing has amassed his or her own collection of listening scenarios. There is always one more story to share from the ever-expanding litany of human experiences requiring a sudden visit to the emergency department.

Storytellers come from the ranks of caregivers. They are passionate about what they want to share with others ([89]). This collection of actual emergency department visits will assist the reader's understanding of the activity and complex equations that are, minute by minute, addressed within their emergency department. Emergency physician and nursing colleagues are invited to add these unique listening lessons to their own quilt-work of emergency department tales.

As caregivers and as 'next of kin', how can we best train our ears to hear? How can we make sure that we are truly listening? How can we practice the optimum translations of each thing we hear and see? Will we pause to remember how easily an initially accepted meaning may turn on a single word, a phrase, an expression, or an added piece of information?

Themes are imbedded within the titles of these stories. This assists recall and retelling. A "Reader's Theater" format ([10]) allows an understandable dialogue to flow when there is a cacophony of multiple voices demanding attention at the same time. It helps the reader listen to who is expressing their thoughts. Each story is different; each patient problem is unique. Each 'next of kin' and each caregiver tries to offer his or her best available assistance. After events unfold there is time to step back and reflect on the immutable shared lessons of the communications in this emergency department visit.   For each story there are a variety of simultaneous tracks being played by the patient, the family and the various caregivers that become involved. Vital signs are important. Identified distractions need to be avoided. The unique canvas that

---

8-10 Medical Literature References

captures this specific emergency department visit can only be completed when each snapshot of the vital history is viewed in the clearest possible focus. Now, to the listening.

1

Just A Virus: Class Trip

Chief Complaint: Left shoulder pain
Emergency department team:
- Dr. Peter
- Dr. Louise
- Dr. John
- Edna
- General Surgery consultant service
- Department volunteer

Communication from:
- Karla (patient)
- Mr. James (father)
- Mrs. James (mother)
- Operating room staff
- Family physician's office

Handover February 25, 23:00
Dr. Peter: Louise, let's start the handover. In A3, we have a fifteen-year-old Karla who presented at 21:00 hours complaining of a sharp pain in her left shoulder followed by nausea and vomiting. She fainted at home before the arrival of the paramedics. They recorded a pulse rate of 130 and blood pressure was 80 over 60. On arrival here, she was looking very pale complaining of severe pain on the top of her left shoulder. John will fill in the details of her history and I will update you on the examination, investigations and management plan.

Dr. John: History is that today Karla had been on a ski trip with her class. She had stopped skiing early because she was tired and the runs were icy. She came back on the school bus and got a ride home with her neighbour. She went to bed without eating supper.

Dr. Peter: Examination revealed a pale fifteen-year-old girl with a very tender left abdomen and shallow respirations. Her rapid pulse and low blood pressure caused concern. She was given a bolus of intravenous fluid as soon as her intravenous line was secured. CAT scan[⊕] has confirmed the ultrasound finding of a fractured spleen[⊕]. She is admitted under the General Surgery service. There are no pediatric intensive care beds. They are looking at increasing staff for a step down bed. The operating room is on alert; operating room personnel are in house. The plan is to observe her very closely, transfuse her to a stable state and avoid surgery, if possible. The surgical service that saw Karla is in the operating room and expects to be there throughout the night.

Dr. John: After an intravenous bolus of a litre of normal saline and the first unit of packed cells[⊕], blood pressure and pulse are already improving.

Dr. Peter: Since she will be with us for a number of hours, I have asked John to keep an eye on her vital signs. He is also obtaining further history from Mr. James, Karla's significantly distressed father.

[⊕] **CAT scan** – computer assisted tomography scan [also **CT scan**]
[⊕] **Fractured spleen** – the breaking of the spleen causing escape of blood into the abdomen
[⊕]**Packed Cells** – blood cells (usually red blood cells) with most of the fluid component removed

Dr. Louise: John let me know if you have any concerns about Karla. Peter, let's review the other patients for handover.

23:30 Main Desk
Dr. Louise: John, give us an update on Karla, the skier with the fractured spleen. Is she stable?

Dr. John: Karla's pulse and blood pressure have stabilized after the two litres of saline and two units of packed red cells. Her haemoglobin was 88. Interesting history…classic! Karla has been home from school for the past week with a sore throat and a lingering cold. Yesterday, her mother took Karla to the family doctor. She had some blood work done. Today was Saturday, and she felt better. This morning, Karla announced to her father that she was going on her school ski trip. Her father, a fire fighter, was just returning home from his midnight shift. Mom had gone off to her twelve-hour shift in the Urgent Care centre, where she is a nurse. Karla and her dad had a big argument when he realized that he had been commissioned to drive her to the school parking lot. She wanted to surprise her other classmates, so she only told her next -door neighbour and asked her to keep it a secret. Dad did not think she should be going if she had not been able to attend school that week. Karla claimed that her doctor had said that it was probably just a virus and she agreed to have "a horrid blood test". Dad relented when the next-door neighbour appeared with her ski gear, ready to join Karla for her promised lift to the school parking lot.

Dr. Louise: Any falls?
Dr. John: None recalled but slipping and sliding all morning on icy runs. Pushed off a large mogul by one of the boys. However, she got up and skied the rest of the

run. Karla was really tired after her lunch and decided to stay in the ski lodge for the afternoon.

Dr. Louise: Anything further on exam?

Dr. John: The improving vital signs and improved colour, as we speak, is reassuring. The chest is clear. The abdomen is diffusely tender to palpation. I didn't want to poke too hard. The rest of the exam shows large tonsils and enlarged nodes in the anterior neck, armpits and groins. I have added a 'monospot'[⊕] to her initial blood work. Edna is comfortable with the fluid and transfusion orders. A second wide-bore intravenous catheter has been secured.

Edna: Dad is finding it hard to forgive himself for not putting his foot down. The two are not exactly talking to each other. The volunteer has offered to arrange a TV and VCR. They are starting to watch the Wizard of Oz from the offered selection of tapes. Dad has a coffee.

Dr. Louise: No better way to share quality time together than a daughter and father listening to the assorted characters found along the yellow brick road of life.

Edna: Karla is getting some of her gusto back. She's explaining to her dad how Dorothy is going to handle 'the know-it-all wizard'. Dad is wisely taking a pass at

---

[⊕] **Monospot (mono test)** – used to help determine whether a person with symptoms has infectious mononucleosis (mono); frequently ordered along with a complete blood count (CBC) which determines whether the number of white blood cells (WBCs) is elevated and whether a significant number of reactive lymphocytes are present; if the mono test is initially negative the doctor may repeat the test one or more weeks later

responding. He just excused himself to find some milk for his coffee.

Dr. John: Karla tells me that Dad is lactose intolerant. Karla recognizes this is Dad's way of saying, "Love you but, at this moment, I don't need to listen to you, girl". I don't think that Karla has realized her next punishment beyond the big needles. Edna has just explained to her that there are to be no visitors and no cell phone until she gets into her own separate room.

Edna: Mom just phoned home and picked up the voice mail messages. Family doctor is reporting a positive mono test and asking to arrange for a follow up visit. Contact precautions with Karla are provided. She should stay home from school for at least two weeks and no sports.

Dr. Louise: Will Karla ever know how close she came to exsanguinating$^{\oplus}$ to death on a ski run or school bus?
Dr. John: No! Maybe! Her mother and father are only too aware.

Dr. Louise: I will give the general surgeon in the operating room a call about the positive mono test. This information may factor into the decision of what parameters he will use in a decision to continue the conservative observation approach or to operate. John, should we put a 'do-not-touch' sign on Karla's abdomen?
Dr. John: A little too late for a sign. It would be interesting to have listened to the conversation that the family doctor had with Karla and her mom. Karla probably did not hear what her mother heard.

$^{\oplus}$**Exsanguinate** – death from massive or continuous blood loss

Edna: I wonder if Mom and Dad took the time to s
the doctor's conversation.

Dr. Louise: I am looking at the admission history
written by the surgical service. Serial vital signs are
recorded but no one addresses the most important
question of the history. Why did this patient rupture her
spleen? At every stage of this patient's illness and
disastrous complication, no one asked "why".

Dr. John: To be fair to Karla, no one knew or thought
to give her the reason why she will be forever considered
one of those individuals who has unnecessarily but
unwittingly risked their life. I think I will have a chat with
Mom, Dad and Karla about how they view the events that
unfolded with Karla today. They may welcome a third
party to help them express their thoughts and fears
regarding the day's events.

ENDNOTES
Chief Complaint – Faint (fifteen-year-old female)
Vital Signs – low blood pressure, rapid pulse, pale
Distractors: parent cross over work shifts, boredom
staying home for a week, 'just a virus', neighbor's arrival,
vital signs, scan results, question of a fall on a ski hill,
quick-tongued teenager.
Snapshots of the vital history:

• A bored teenage daughter challenges a tired
parent.

• Viruses have consequences.

• Did the family doctor convey the presumptive
diagnosis of the Infectious Mononucleosis[⊕]?

[⊕]**Mononucleosis** – usually caused by the Epstein-Barr virus (EBV); a general
malaise followed by a set of signs and symptoms that may include high fever,
severe sore throat, swelling of the lymph nodes, fatigue loss of appetite,
muscle aches, enlargement of the spleen, swollen tonsils, and mild jaundice

mother share the presumptive diagnosis
?

there any instructions about contact and
ʌutions?

the abdomen examined for an enlarged
ʌusual lymph nodes?

ɪd the surgeons consider the background cause
of the fractured spleen?

- Was this emergency avoidable?
- Does the patient know how she had inadvertently put her life in danger?
- Can the parents forgive themselves?
- Is this a good time to offer a listening ear to the family members?

The stage is set. Karla was bored. The fifteen-year-old was determined not to miss a class ski trip after spending a week at home. The parents were working on opposite shifts. Twenty-four hours previous, the family doctor did not spell out any concerns or precautions. Was the adenopathy[⊕] and enlarged spleen not detectable? Did the surgical caregivers translate all of these physical findings and the vital history? A young life was put at risk. The vital history has revealed itself. Karla knows the role she played and the inadvertent risk she took. It is a good time to offer a listening ear to Karla and her parents.

⊕ **Adenopathy** – swollen lymph glands

2

Two Fathers Notified: No One Listens

Chief Complaint: DOA$^{\oplus}$
Emergency department team:
- Dr. Peter
- Dr. Louise
- Edward
- Ward clerk
- Dr. John
- Social worker

Communication from:
- Medical coroner$^{\oplus}$
- Dr. Bill Smith

Failed communication:
- Two sons with two fathers

Handover February 27, 16:00

Dr. Peter: Louise, I have written down a log of the status of each patient in sections A, B and C. We don't have anyone from section D to hand over. Triage$^{\oplus}$has eight patients. There is an eighteen-year-old accident victim from an all-terrain vehicle. He has been intubated

---

$^{\oplus}$ **DOA** – Dead On Arrival

$^{\oplus}$ **Coroner** – a government official (usually a qualified physician) who investigates, confirms and certifies the occurrence and the cause of death of an individual within a jurisdiction

$^{\oplus}$ **Triage** – an accepted organized system of categorizing relative urgency of patient injuries/symptoms/signs and delineating the proscribed order to attend to or re-assess these injuries or symptoms

in the field. The trauma team is expecting his arrival in ten minutes. I will just provide you with a heads up on the activity around the interview rooms where you see the police officers and a number of people milling around. The medical coroner has arrived and is talking to family members of the twenty-four-year-old male who has been missing for two weeks. A body has been found matching the description. Mother, father and sister are waiting to be taken to the hospital morgue to identify the body. More family members are arriving each minute.

Edward: Peter, the ward clerk has a Dr. Bill Smith on the line. You need to talk to him. He wants to send us a fifty-year-old male with acute agitated depression. He wants you to see him and give him something to calm him down.

Dr. Louise: I will take the call if you and John are finished with the handover.

Edward: Louise, you need to talk to him now. You need to say "No"! Tell him the charge nurse says that he can't send his patient here.

Dr. Louise: Hi Bill, Louise here, I have just taken over for Peter. What's up?

Dr. Bill: Hi Louise. I have a difficult problem here in my office. James is a fifty-year-old man whom I am worried about. He continues bursts of shouting and punching the wall. Not much I can garner from him. There are utterances about police and about his son. It would seem that his son has been arrested. He can't control his grief and his anger. I am sending him to your emergency department. Can you give him a tranquilizer and possibly get Psychiatry to see him? He will likely need admission.

Dr. Louise: Not good Bill. You can't send him here.

Dr. Bill: Why not? You are just across the street from us.

Dr. Louise: The situation here is that the case of the missing twenty-four-year-old male from these past two past weeks is now unravelling. A body has been found. A murder investigation is underway. The body has just arrived at our morgue. The coroner is taking the parents to identify the body. Police have arrested a twenty-year-old male. The social worker is talking to an expanding number of family members who are arriving in our waiting room.

Dr. Bill: What can I do with him here?

Dr. Louise: My advice is to absolutely not direct him here. See if you can find family members to come in to assist you. If you decide that you need him assessed for self-harm call the psychiatry service at the other hospital.

Dr. Bill: But we're just across the street from you.

Dr. Louise: Yes, and just a few feet from a family that is likely to turn into a mob seeking revenge for the murder of a young family member. If necessary, you can call EMS to help with the transfer. They may ask for police escort. I will let the ambulance dispatch know so that they understand about not transporting him to the nearest hospital. If you are otherwise worried, I can ask one of the officers here to come to your office.

Handover February 28, 16:00

Dr. Peter: Louise, I may have left you with a difficult problem yesterday. I had not picked up on Edward's message that, "You need to say no!" Did you get through to Bill?

Dr. Louise: I think so. His patient was seen at the other hospital and arrangements were made for admission. Yesterday, our emergency department was the crossroad to a forever changed tomorrow for two families. Two fathers, of the murdered twenty-four-year-old male and the arrested twenty-year-old male, did not want to listen to what they did not want to hear. John and Edward were just filling us in on the story that's gone somewhat public today.

Dr. Peter: Tell us the latest story on the street.

Dr. John: The murder investigation is for Steven, the twenty-four-year-old male whose body was identified by his parents yesterday in our morgue. Steven had had no communication with his parents for some three years. He lived in a neighbouring community. A month ago, his sister had shared her suspicion that their mother was hooked on amphetamines and getting them from a known drug dealer. Steven had set up surveillance and surreptitiously made a video recording of the dealer extorting money from his mother.

Dr. Peter: What was the father's take on the daughter's concern?

Dr. John: The father was unaware of anything being amiss. He was completing a six-month posting at the military base some two hundred kilometres away. Steven had phoned him to discuss the concerns he had about his mother. The father had refused to talk to Steven about his children's suspicions of the mother's drug use. A few nights later, Steven apparently confronted the drug dealer in a bar and threatened to turn over the video to police if he did not stop selling drugs to his mother. Later that week, Steven's place of employment noted his absence for two consecutive days. The sister was his 'next of kin' contact. There was significant evidence of a search and destroy rampage within Steven's apartment. Next day, the police started a missing person investigation. After repeated questioning over two days the sister revealed to police the concern she had shared with her brother about their mother. The daughter and the mother were asked to review random pictures of individuals who might have been seen around the parents' house. Police recorded their facial and verbal responses to the recognition questions. Mother finally broke down and named one of the individuals in the photos. Police knew him as a drug peddler with multiple minor skirmishes at bars and one conviction for possession of stolen goods. They arranged phone tapping and surveillance. The surveillance team noted that on two occasions, while driving on snow covered Concession Road 5, their suspect slowed down to almost a stop.

Edward: Yesterday a group of officers combed the nearby wooded field. They found the body in a ravine behind a dense strand of trees and a lot of trampled snow and snowmobile tracks. They got a search warrant for the drug dealer's home and car. They found a rifle in his trunk. On checking, they noted that it matched the description of the rifle that his own father had reported stolen from his truck some two weeks previous.

Dr. John: The son apparently told his father that the rifle had disappeared from his father's truck when he borrowed it to move some furniture. He had asked his father not to report the theft to police because he thought that he knew who had taken it and he would be able to get it back in a few days or a week.

Dr. Peter: No one was willing to listen to anyone. Family members also held back information from the police. Secrecy and crime was more important than listening. One can see how the police were hampered in their efforts to assist. Even doctors don't want to listen to facts that complicate their day.

ENDNOTES
Chief Complaint – DOA (twenty-four-year-old male)
Vital Signs – absent
Distractors: poor family communications, withheld information
Snapshots of the vital history:
- Two families are devastated by a refusal to listen.
- No one wants to listen to what they do not want to hear.
- A refusal to listen carries an immeasurable risk.
- Why did the victim's father refuse to listen to his son?
- Why did the assailant's father not listen to his son?
- Why did the daughter hold back information from the police?
- Why did the mother hold back information from the police?
- Why did the family doctor object to the refusal of accepting a transfer?
- Was this death avoidable?
- Does the future hold any likelihood of enhanced listening within the two families?

Histories collide. After three years of non-communication did the father of the murder victim think that the request for dialogue concerning the mother's health was frivolous? Why did the father of the suspected assailant go to police instead of questioning his son about the misplaced rifle? Both mother and sister withhold valuable information from the police. Everyone has his or her own convenient agenda. Sometimes we can only look on and wonder.

3

Accusing Glances: Not Guilty

Chief Complaint: Broken arm
Emergency department team:
- Dr. Peter
- Dr. Louise
- Edna
- Dr. John
- Triage nurse
- Department volunteer
- X-ray technician
- 'On-duty' professional staff

Patient: Thomas
Communication with:
- Mrs. James (mother of Thomas)
- Mr. James (father and patient)

Handover March 15, 20:00
Dr. Peter: Louise, I have written down a log of the status of each patient in sections A through D. Beyond the call of the grim reaper, we are told that there are no inpatient beds. There is also a massive stroke that won't survive the coming morning. DNR$^{\oplus}$ details are known and the charge nurse is looking for a more family conducive

---

$^{\oplus}$ **DNR** – Do Not Resuscitate

surrounding. Triage⊕ has eight patients. No known transfers expected.

Edna: Peter, there are two further patients that have been registered under you but you have not seen them. Should I switch them to Louise?

Dr. Peter: Yes, please, what is their problem?

Edna: Tag team of father and son. James is the thirty-year-old father who fainted at triage. Thomas is his two-year-old son who is waiting for an x-ray for a possible broken arm.

Dr. Louise: How did he break his arm?

Edna: John, you took the history from the triage nurse.

Dr. John: Thomas, the child, was playing in the bathtub. He slipped and Dad caught him by the wrist just as his head hit the water. There was a sudden loud, shrill scream. Now he won't use his arm. Thomas has been crying for the last hour.

Dr. Louise: How did Dad get hurt? Why did they call you to triage?

Dr. John: This is the second visit for a broken arm for Thomas. Father got quite agitated with the nurse's questions at the triage desk. A few minutes later he suddenly slipped off the chair and onto the floor. A volunteer saw the slide occurring and quickly grabbed Thomas as Dad rolled onto the floor. I was called to assess

---

⊕ **Triage** – an accepted organized system of categorizing relative urgency of patient injuries/symptoms/signs and delineating the proscribed order to attend to or re-assess these injuries or symptoms

the father who is now on a stretcher in D4. His initial vital signs were normal and they are being repeated. No seizure activity. His glucometer$^\oplus$ recording was normal.

Dr. Louise: Where is Thomas?

Edna: The volunteer has the baby. Thomas won't use his right arm.

Dr. Louise: Did anyone examine his arm?

Dr. John: No use! He cries anywhere you touch him. Triage completed a requisition for an x-ray of the right arm.

Edna: The x-ray technician wants to know what part to x-ray.

Dr. Louise: John, let's go find this train wreck. What do you think may be wrong with Thomas?

Dr. John: Many things are possible with a crying two-year-old.

20:15 – Bedside Thomas
Dr. Louise: Good, Mom is here now. Mrs. James, I am Dr. Louise and this is Dr. John, our emergency medicine resident, who has been busy checking out Dad after he fainted at triage. We will check Mr. James again. First, let's have a good look at Thomas. We are told that he fell in the bathtub. Mom, can you sit in this chair and hold Thomas in your lap with his back against you and Thomas facing us? Now, can you wrap your arms completely

---

$^\oplus$ **Glucometer** – measuring instrument for 'stat (immediate)' blood glucose (sugar) level

around his left arm and his trunk and have him sit straight up on your lap? I suspect that there may not be a broken arm but we need to play with Thomas for a few moments just touching and checking different parts of his right arm while you hold him still in your lap. John, go ahead and identify your findings. Examine the least likely areas of injury first and then proceed to the next most likely area of injury in a two-year-old child.

Dr. John: Collarbone...no added grief. Wrist and fingers...no added grief. Shoulder...no added grief. Thomas doesn't like my touching his elbow and Thomas won't show me the palm of his hand when I try to get him to hold onto the tongue depressor.

Dr. Louise: Mom, Dr. John is going to pull up a chair and sit in front of and facing Thomas. He will manipulate the elbow joint. Thomas is certainly going to scream but it will only last for one to two seconds. After John completes the procedure we expect that Thomas will start using his arm again within a minute. John, it is important that, after you position both of your hands, you do the manoeuvre through the entire proscribed range of movement. If you stop, Thomas will wriggle away from you and Mom will run away with Thomas. The entire manoeuvre should last no longer than ten seconds.

Dr. John: Seven seconds and I certainly heard and felt the click.

Edna: The scream was louder!
Dr. Louise: Done, Thomas! Mom, Thomas doesn't like us and he may not want to see us ever again. I expect he will start using the arm in a few minutes. Let's see what Dad is up to.

Dr. John: Dad, you probably heard the scream. This is Dr. Louise, my staff attending emergency physician.

20:20 – Bedside Mr. James

Dr. Louise: Hi Dad, Thomas probably doesn't have a broken arm. He just slipped one of the ligaments at his elbow. It is called 'nursemaid's elbow'. We think it's back in place now. There he is. He wants to come and see you but he's rather wary of big bad John standing in his way. Mom and Dad, I have to tell you that this can happen again.

Mr. James: When?

Dr. Louise: Anytime. Especially in the next two years—less as he gets older.

Mrs. James: Why did it happen?

Dr. Louise: What causes it most often is a twisting motion from above. The situation usually occurs when young children try to get away from your grasp, especially when putting on winter clothing.

Mr. James: I don't think I can bear the thought of having to face the suspicious glances I received at triage when I brought Thomas in. I must look like a child abuser—I will never forget the fixated beam in the eyes of that nurse. I was guilty! Guilty!

Dr. Louise: When children are hurt, moms and especially dads interpret each pointed glance and direct question from triage and throughout the emergency department as fully loaded with suspicion. Mr. James, you were probably feeling a little guilty for letting Thomas play a bit too boisterously in the tub. You grabbed him reflexively. That happens a lot in the bathroom, probably every evening. It is akin to winding up a toy seal and asking it not to do tricks. Plus, Mom wants you to use lots of soap. That makes them even more slippery.

Dr. John: A second factor is that your son's chart shows that Thomas has had a greenstick fracture$^{\oplus}$ a few months ago. Thomas is going to be a challenge for you and for us for some time.

Mr. James: Tell me about it!

Dr. Louise: Dad and Mom, you need to be prepared to be alert to a more significant suspicion that may be cast against you. That is the bruise seen on your son's lower back.

Mrs. James: That is—

Dr. Louise: First, let me explain. In this part of the country, our staff may get to see that kind of 'bruise' only once or twice in a professional career.

Mr. James: But it is not a bruise. It is permanent. He was born with it.

Dr. Louise: Can I ask both of you to do us a big favour?

Mr. James: What are you asking?

Dr. Louise: While we reassess you, I would like our volunteer to show off Thomas with a romp around the

---

$^{\oplus}$ **Greenstick fracture** – a break in a long bone (usually a child's) where the bark of the bone is buckled but there is no gap at the fracture site

department asking Thomas to give a goodbye 'high-five' to each of the nursing and resident physician staff. We will arrange to keep his pyjama bottoms purposely hung low. Dr. John will follow and record, from each member of the staff, their opinion of the noticed discoloration. John, there are to be no hints and no offering of any other available information. The tour and repeated 'high-fives' will also help convince Mom and Dad that Thomas doesn't need to have an x-ray for what is not a broken arm.

20:35 – Bedside Mr. James

Dr. Louise: The results are in. First, Dad has a bruise under his bald spot. Second, Dad is not guilty. Third, Thomas is 'a ham' who won't soon be forgotten. He will definitely be talked up among the staff and yes, also a few patients and their families. Dr. John, give us the survey results.

Dr. John: Four said that it was a bruise from a fall, six don't know, two thought it was a blood disorder and one correctly identified it as a 'Mongolian spot'[⊕].

[⊕] **Mongolian spot** – flat blue or gray birthmarks on a newborn or child most commonly located on lower back and buttocks; although they can look like bruises, they are normal and not a sign of child abuse or any other condition

[⊕] **Mongolian spot** – flat blue or gray birthmarks on a newborn or child most commonly located on lower back and buttocks; although they can look like bruises, they are normal and not a sign of child abuse or any other condition

Dr. Louise: John, Edna reports that the correct answer (Mongolian Spot$^{\oplus}$) came from you. We congratulate you on your efficient use of Google. Good night, Thomas. We know you'll come back to visit us again. Slow down a little bit for Dad's sake. Thanks to you, Mom and Dad. A happy child at play can provide us with a lot of valuable information.

Edna: All too often, parents and caregivers respond to a crying child with an abundance of suspicion and imagine 'worst case scenarios'.

Handover March 18, 08:00
Dr. Louise: Has everyone seen the thank you card from 'Thomas the Bruiser'? John, Thomas will certainly remember you.

Edna: Loudest scream anyone in this department has had to hear in a while.

Dr. John: I understand now how unfair it is to order an x-ray without focusing on what information you are seeking.

Dr. Louise: The evening bath ritual often produces a few tears. Sometimes from the parent!

Edna: Sometimes the parent finds it impossible to control the chaos.

ENDNOTES

Chief Complaint -- Broken arm (two–year-old boy)

Vital Signs -- uncontrolled crying

Distractions: bath time, crying child, past history of arm fracture, fainting father, unusual bruise.

Snapshots of the vital history:

- A second occurrence of a broken arm in a child brings accusatory glances at triage.
- The emergency department is a questioning environment.
- A father blames himself for his son's injury.
- Volunteers are indispensable to care and teaching.
- There is a 'look-up' role for Google.
- Why do we always jump to our first conclusions?
- Can a caregiver's face and body language cast accusation?
- Do caregivers and 'next of kin' trust each other?
- Was the father's faint and injury avoidable?
- Can we picture the scene in the bathroom?
- Can children at play modify our translations of what we see and hear?

The emergency department is a questioning environment. Accusatory questions and glances are cast when a two-year-old presents with a broken arm for the second time. What about the bruise on the child's back? Does this father feel guilty? How will he be judged?

4

Forgotten Convenience: Unexpected Visitors

Chief Complaint: Leg pain
Emergency department team:
- Dr. Peter
- Dr. Louise
- Dr. John
- Edward
- Orthopaedic consultants
- Radiology consultant

Communication with:
- Harvey (patient)
- Mrs. James (mother)

Handover May 05; 16:00

Dr. Peter: Louise, I will review with you the status of each patient in each section. John and I will be here for a while finishing up on some of these cases. First, we want to tell you about one patient that has presented somewhat of an enigma and has caused John and I to fall behind today.

Dr. Louise: Looks like you've had a busy Sunday shift.

Dr. Peter: In A1, we have Harvey, a twenty-year-old university student who came in by ambulance screaming about pain in his left butt and thigh. Harvey was in the triathlon this morning. Pain started halfway through his run. He couldn't finish. He arrived by ambulance. The pain has steadily increased even after receiving 15 milligrams of morphine over thirty minutes. He arrived with a pulse of 110 and a blood pressure 140 over 80. He has normal distal pulses and capillary refill. His temperature is normal.

Dr. Louise: Are there any findings on exam?

Dr. John: There's no swelling or discoloration or bruising anywhere. His buttocks, hamstrings and quads are very tight and tender to any palpation. His abdomen is benign. Chest is clear. All distal pulses are palpable.

Dr. Peter: Mrs. James, his mother is somewhat overwhelmed by her son's agony. There is no past history of swelling or injury. There are no abnormalities in sensation, movement or reflexes of upper or lower extremities. John has tried, once again, to clarify any pertinent past history.

Dr. John: Harvey arrived unannounced at his mother's place with two university friends yesterday afternoon. It took them three hours to get there by car. Last evening, they signed up for today's triathlon as a team with Harvey being designated to do the run. They went out for supper and returned by 9 p.m. The mother arranged some cots and blankets for them in the basement where they crashed before midnight. They left for the downtown start before seven this morning.

Dr. Louise: Any alcohol? Any medication? Any drug use? Any sports enhancing drugs? Any evidence of skin puncture? Any skin discoloration?

Dr. John: No, to each of those questions. No falls and no injuries recalled. All three of them have each previously completed individual triathlons. They are somewhat 'out of shape' this year and decided to enter as a team. Harvey opted for the 'run portion'. Late last night, Harvey had asked his mom for some of her arthritis medicine because his hamstrings were a little tight from the long car ride. Mom didn't have any. Harvey found some aspirin in the bathroom cabinet and said that would suffice.

Dr. Peter: The light drizzle and cool temperatures certainly would not make you think that heat had anything to do with this presentation. What investigations have you been able to manage so far?

Dr. John: X-ray of the pelvis, hips and femurs reveal no abnormality. An ultrasound does not suggest deep vein thrombosis. We've sent off some blood work including type and cross and blood cultures. We have also asked for a stat consult from the orthopaedic service. I'll accompany Edward who is taking Harvey to CAT scan. We will need some more morphine. He has a second intravenous line started even though his blood pressure remains stable. Any further suggestions?

Dr. Peter: Check if there has been any fever or viral illness in the preceding week? Ask about family history of muscle problems and any travel out of the country. Ask about any recollection of eating raw or undercooked meat. Go ahead and we will check the blood results as they come up on the screen.

Dr. Louise: The initial blood work is unremarkable except for kidney function; his elevated creatinine$^{\oplus}$ level confirms significant kidney dysfunction. Peter was there any flank pain or tenderness?

Dr. Peter: No! Edward, did John check the urine?

Edward: No, I dipped it and it was positive for blood. John said that that would not be too unusual a finding after a long run.

Dr. Peter: Are we sure it is blood?

Edward: What do you mean?

Dr. Peter: Let me spin the urine and I will look for blood cells under the microscope.

16:30 Main Desk (Louise, Edward and Peter)
Dr. Louise: John is calling from the CAT scan unit. The initial reporting does not show any suggestion of an avulsion fracture or any other bony abnormality. There's no evidence of muscle hematoma or muscle abscess or air in the tissues. However, the muscles are very swollen and tight within their compartments. The radiologist is suggesting that the Orthopedic surgeons$^{\oplus}$ may want to measure the pressure within these compartments. What did the orthopods say when they examined Harvey?

$^{\oplus}$ **Creatinine** – a blood test, which is used to evaluate kidney function; a by-product of creatine, which is involved with muscle energy metabolism; filtered from the blood by the kidneys and excreted into urine
$^{\oplus}$ **Orthopedic Surgery** _ Specialty concerned with bony skeleton, joints and muscles (also – **Orthopods** and **Orthopedic service**)

Edward: They are on their way to look at the CAT scan with the radiologist. They are concerned that, on their examination, both buttocks and both thighs are very tender and quite rock hard. They are talking about taking him to the operating room.

Dr. Peter: Louise and Edward, there are no red blood cells in the spun and unspun urine. I am going to repeat the blood work and add another set of blood cultures, lactic acid, arterial blood gas$^{\oplus}$ and a serum myoglobin$^{\oplus}$. It is reasonable to send the urine for a drug screen.

17:20

Dr. Louise: I will call the ICU resident and staff to free an ICU bed and to help us calculate further massive intravenous fluids, establish a central line and an arterial line here or in the operating room. Peter, for now, do you agree to a bolus of 2 litres of normal saline wide open?

Dr. Peter: Yes, let's crosscheck the calculation for the initial bicarbonate dose. We may need to ask Nephrology$^{\oplus}$ about dialysis.

Dr. Louise: I will remind John to ask Harvey again about any drugs or medications. I will repeat the same query with his mother and his friends.

$^{\oplus}$ **Arterial Blood Gas** – sample of blood from an artery for the measurement of acid base balance (pH and the concentration of oxygen, carbon dioxide and bicarbonate]

$^{\oplus}$**Myoglobin** - – the special protein in muscle cells

$^{\oplus}$ **Nephrology** – the specialty for kidney disorders

17:30 Bedside Harvey

Dr. Peter: Mrs. James, within the next hour, the orthopaedic surgeons are arranging to take Harvey to the operating room. They need to open up the envelopes surrounding Harvey's leg muscles. The individual muscle cells of his butt and upper legs are extremely swollen. As they continue to swell, they burst, releasing their contents outside the cell walls and increasing the pressure in the envelopes surrounding the muscle groups. From what, we don't know, but if allowed to continue, the blood supply to all of the muscles in the legs will be cut off.

Mrs. James: Is there anything I can do?

Dr. Peter: There is one further thing that should be done. Ask Harvey's friends to go back to the house and give them permission to search through all of Harvey's clothes, shaving kit and your bathroom cabinets and for anything that looks like pills or powder and bring back to us anything they find.

Handover May 07, 16:00

Dr. Louise: Peter and John, a follow up on the case you handed over two days ago. Harvey has had a rocky forty-eight hours. Diagnosis was diffuse rhabdomyolysis[⊕]. Literally there was a signal for all of the active skeletal muscle cells to break down and spill their myoglobin protein outside the cell walls. The most active exercising muscles fared the worst fate. Harvey's serum myoglobin level was astronomical. He had all of his leg compartments opened surgically with repeat operating room assessment of each compartment twenty-four hours

---

[⊕] **Rhabdomyolysis** – a breakdown of muscle cells emptying their contents into the blood circulation and into the rigid envelope covering of the specific involved muscle(s)

later. He received massive amounts of intravenous fluids. His creatinine$^{⊕}$ rise seems to have plateaued this morning. His kidney function has not worsened. That points to recovery. Dialysis is not being planned.

Dr. John: What was the cause?

Dr. Louise: Extreme exercise plus something else. The urine drug screen was negative. After the operating room, the mother remembered that the aspirin that Harvey said he took for his hamstring tightness likely was not aspirin but the mother's anti-lipid medication. The mother had put a half dozen of them in the empty aspirin bottle when she went to an out-of-town conference last spring. She recalls that there were still three or four pills left, and she had left them in the same container for future out of town trips.

Dr. Peter: I imagine that the mother is having a hard time realizing that her simple act of convenience could have brought such devastating consequences to her son.

Dr. Louise: Harvey did not even know that his mother had started an anti-lipid medication two years ago.

Dr. John: She's probably not consoled by the fact that the occurrence of anti-lipids causing rhabdomyolysis is extremely rare.

ENDNOTES
Chief Complaint – Severe leg pain (twenty-year-old male)

$^{⊕}$ **Creatinine** – a blood test, which is used to evaluate kidney function; a by-product of creatine, which is involved with muscle energy metabolism; filtered from the blood by the kidneys and excreted into urine

Vital Signs – within normal limits considering the excruciating pain

Distractions: unexpected visit, severity of pain, location of pain, triathlon run, onset time

Snapshots of the vital history:

- Failure to recall an act of convenience can have serious consequences.

- Severe pain without an identifiable cause poses a challenge.

- Caregivers must rule out initial diagnostic assumptions.

- The vital history holds the clue that will determine both the diagnosis and the cause.

- Early consultation allows for quick response to therapeutic procedures.

- Quick action is needed to avoid catastrophe.

- Do we know what medications our parents/housemates take?

- Do we always read the brochure before we take a medication?

- Do we know how to identify a simple 'aspirin' tablet?

- Are we always certain about the medications we are taking?

- When is blood in the urine not blood in the urine?

When a standard approach to diagnosis and investigation of sudden severe pain reveals no leads, there are only two directions the diagnostic pendulum can swing: advanced testing or a more detailed vital history. The recollection of a mother's act of convenience is delayed but is sufficient to confirm an unexpected causation. The initial presumed finding of blood within the urine sample requires correction in light of the other history and investigative findings. Early consultation, quick investigation and aggressive treatment modalities are unleashed.

5

My Daughter Always Faints: Listen

Chief Complaint: Faint
Emergency department team:
- School teacher
- Paramedics
- Dr. Louise
- Dr. Peter
- Edna
- Dr. John
- Pediatric resident
- Cardiology resident

Communication with:
- Margaret (patient)
- Mr. James (father)

Handover June 02, 14:00

Dr. Peter: Thanks for coming in early today, Louise. I have just reviewed each section and all of the patients are admitted or awaiting discharge with orders completed for each. Radiology reported a missed undisplaced wrist fracture in a fourteen-year-old. Talked to Mom on the phone; she will bring him back for a cast this evening. The only remaining patient for handover today is Margaret, a thirteen-year-old girl who collapsed at school, was given CPR⊕ on site and brought here by ambulance. On arrival, she was fully alert and had normal vital signs.

⊕ **CPR** – cardio-pulmonary resuscitation

Edna: John is in A2 doing the work-up on Margaret. I think that may be her father being directed by the triage nurse to our desk.

Dr. Peter: Mr. James, I am Dr. Peter and this is Dr. Louise who is taking over as the attending physician. Margaret seems fine. She is in the second room to the right. Dr. John, the emergency medicine resident, is in the room trying to further assess what happened at school. Edna, the emergency nurse, is on her way there, too. Dr. John is coming out so you can follow Edna to Margaret's room.

Mr. James: Why did they bring her here? Margaret faints all the time.

Dr. Peter: Louise, since John has got the initial details and completed the initial assessment, I will ask him to complete the handover for Margaret. John let us in on the history; her dad says she faints all the time. Why did they call the ambulance? Why did they bring Margaret here?

Dr. John: History from the paramedics is that Margaret is a thirteen-year-old girl who was sitting on a chair in her grade eight classroom when she suddenly fell to the floor. After a ten second loss of consciousness, the teacher was not able to obtain a pulse. The teacher started CPR. A classmate used the teacher's cell phone to call 911. After thirty seconds Margaret took a gasp. By the time the paramedics arrived, Margaret was asking, "What happened?" The paramedics recorded normal vital signs at the scene. She may have had a fainting spell and the pulse was too slow or too weak for detection. Her vital signs remained stable during transport.

Dr. Peter: John, Dad has told us that this has happened a number of times.

Dr. John: Margaret doesn't recall the events but she has been told about them. She blacks out or faints and then she is back to normal. The family doctor saw her last week and referred her to the pediatric clinic. Her appointment is this week. She reports that she has had blood work and an ECG done. She is not aware of any concerns of seizure. She was questioned about her sports activity and her periods. There is no known family history of faints or seizures. She does not experience a warning aura and she is unaware of the episode coming on. She just wakes up on the floor or the ground. To date, there have been no significant injuries with the falls. She feels a little fuzzy for a minute but does not complain of headaches. There has been no evidence of tongue biting or incontinence with any of the episodes.

Dr. Louise: How many episodes?

Dr. John: Margaret thinks about six events in total but she hasn't told her parents each time she has suspected an occurrence, because she is not sure if she has had one when no one else is around. She is also embarrassed to mention it.

Dr. Louise: Anything on examination?
Dr. John: Margaret is tall for her thirteen years. She is fully alert and oriented in time, person and place. Her only complaint is a sore lower anterior chest. Breath sounds are normal. The abdomen is soft and the neurological

examination is completely normal. Listening to her heart sounds reveals a 'grade three pan-systolic$^{\oplus}$ murmur'.

Dr. Louise: What does the ECG show?

Dr. John: The monitor shows a regular rhythm at a rate of 74. ECG shows what could be a right or a partial left bundle branch block. The presence of left ventricular hypertrophy$^{\oplus}$ is hard to judge with the bundle branch and her age.

Edna: The glucometer reading is within normal limits.

14:15 Bedside Margaret
Mr. James: Can I take her home now? Margaret seems to be hungry.

Dr. Louise: Dad, from what Dr. John has told us, we should keep Margaret for a few hours, monitor her heart rhythm and run some other tests. We will also ask our cardiology$^{\oplus}$ and pediatric$^{\oplus}$ colleagues to see her. What do you make of these episodes Margaret is having?

Mr. James: Margaret is otherwise healthy, not one for sports, but can beat up her fourteen-year-old brother. She has had three episodes witnessed by family members in the past two months. The family doctor saw her two weeks ago. She was asked about her diet and about starting her periods. There is an appointment scheduled with the pediatric clinic this week. I think she may have

---

$^{\oplus}$ **Pan-systolic** – the entire time period spanning the first to the second heart sound

$^{\oplus}$ **Ventricular Hypertrophy** – overly enlarged main muscle mass of the heart (left or right or both)

$^{\oplus}$ **Cardiology** – Specialty for heart disorders

$^{\oplus}$ **Pediatrics** – Specialty for children disorders

had more episodes, but whenever we ask, she says no. I have only witnessed one episode. Last year, she fainted on the dock at the cottage and fell into the water. Thought she was just fooling but when I pulled her out of the water she was lifeless. Then she coughed and seemed to come around. We should have brought her in to the hospital but she was fine in every way.

Dr. John: Does Margaret ever complain of pain in her chest, back, head, arms or legs?

Mr. James: No.

Dr. John: Does she ever have unexplained episodes of shortness of breath or sweating?

Mr. James: Not that she has mentioned. She doesn't like sports. She feels she is too clumsy.

Dr. Peter: John noted that there was no family history for early heart disease or seizures. Is that correct?

Mr. James: The only talk of seizures in the family, especially because of Margaret's fainting spells, has been when my sister died from drowning in her backyard pool.

Dr. Peter: Have any other family members experienced faints, loss of consciousness or early, unexpected accidental death?

Mr. James: I recall a cousin who fell out of a tree and died when we were about ten years old. We were always told that he had broken his neck in the fall.

15:30 Main Desk

Dr. Louise: Peter before you leave, John has an update for you on Margaret, today's young fainter. Interesting! The cardiac echo shows sub-aortic hypertrophic cardiomyopathy[⊕]. After much debate, Pediatrics and Cardiology settled on the location of the best admission ward for Margaret. Pediatrics and Cardiology plan to give grand rounds on Margaret in two weeks. Cardiology is arranging to address the roles of internal pacemakers and implantable defibrillators in these patients. Cardiac Surgery will be asked to discuss the experience with surgical coring of the hypertrophied heart muscle. Pediatrics and Emergency will discuss presenting symptoms that could suggest the diagnosis. We also plan to send out an electronic poster to invite the participation of all of our professional hospital staff and interested community nurses and physicians.

Dr. John: It was hard to accept the possibility of a serious life-threatening event having occurred in Margaret when she seemed to be just fine. The background history provided by Margaret's father was undeniably suggestive of an ominous problem. The ECG findings suggested the possibility of a heart anomaly. At first listen to the heart sounds, I was still discounting the loudness of the murmur to her thin body habitus. When I listen now, the murmur is undeniably very loud and abnormal.

Dr. Louise: John, let's ask the Pediatric and Cardiology residents if they can do an audiogram of

---

[⊕] **Sub-Aortic Hypertrophic Cardiomyopathy** – a genetic familial disorder where the left ventricular muscle mass under the aortic valve is significantly hypertrophied resulting in flow diminution and lethal arrhythmia;
Arrhythmia – abnormal heart beats in terms of rate and/or regularity

Margaret's heart sounds. It is understandable that everyone wants to listen to the murmur. It will become more than a little overwhelming to Margaret to face a mounting line-up of 'listeners'. They could use the special stethoscope in the teleconference suite. The audio recording could also be used to open up the case presentation.

Dr. Peter: Great pick up, John. In a logical manner, you pursued a presentation that made no sense and arrived at a diagnosis that needs action. You may want to check with Mom and Dad and do a family tree. DNA$^{\oplus}$ testing for the offending dominant gene is now available. The transmission of the specific faulty gene from one of the parents' accounts for more than half of the recognized cases. The remaining cases come from 'de novo' gene mutations. Family history of young deaths in this syndrome is often masked by the attribution to accidental causes. Autopsy is usually not requested when there is a reasonable accidental cause for the death. It is important to listen to each of their stories and to do the initial ECG and Cardiac Echo screening tests.

Dr. John: Dad is overwhelmed right now, but I did mention workups for individual family members. I gave him our names and asked permission to call him next week. When I left him, Dad was calling Margaret's teacher who had left her phone number with the ward clerk. He wanted to call her to express his gratitude for her quick action. I will also ask Margaret and her father for permission to complete an audiogram recording.

$^{\oplus}$ **DNA** – deoxyribonucleic acid; responsible for storing and transferring genetic information

Edna: Tell Dad not to forget that Margaret is still hungry.

ENDNOTES
Chief Complaint – Faint (thirteen-year-old girl)
Vital Signs – normal
Distractions: normal vital signs from EMS[⊕] at school, recent doctor assessment
Snapshots of the vital history:

- A history of recurrent faints needs a full workup.
- Rare diagnostic cases need to be shared with all caregivers.
- Can children have cardiac arrests?
- Potentially affected family members need to be assessed.
- Are relatives at risk for sudden death?
- Can we reduce the bright light of notoriety focussing on a young girl?
- Do we sometimes forget to thank the 'first responder'?
- What is the prognosis for this patient?

The search for involved family members at risk of sudden death will multiply the gains beyond Margaret. The history and the heart sounds give the same message. The first responder's successful resuscitation began the translation of what listening was needed. Although mind boggling, the employed protective devices are lifesaving over and over again.

[⊕] **EMS** – emergency medical services

6

Luke's Bear: A Family's Loss

Chief Complaint: Trauma Team
Emergency department team:
- Dr. Louise
- Dr. Peter
- Dr. John
- Edna
- Ward clerk
- Staff general surgeon
- Anaesthesiology consultant
- Respiratory therapist
- Dr. Susan (trauma team leader)
- Neurosurgeon consultant
- Radiology consultant
- Registration clerk
- Senior pediatric resident
- Orthopaedic consultant

Patients: Marian (mother); Janet (daughter)
Communication with:
- James Knight (father)
- Police officer
- Tom (uncle)
- Catherine (grandmother)
- Luke (son)

Handover July 03, 15:00
Dr. Louise: Peter, are you ready for handover?

Dr. Peter: As ready as I'll ever be! It's the long weekend and there are two serious trauma patients that have occupied most of our attention over the past hour. Welcome to a brand new crop of residents. This was a true baptism by fire for the novice members of the trauma team. In trauma bay A1 there was a thirty-something female who apparently rolled an open jeep on County Road 7. She was extricated from under the car with a coma scale of 6 out of 15. She was intubated at the scene and on arrival here had a systolic blood pressure of 100, a pulse of 80 and a fixed dilated left pupil. No other obvious life threatening injuries. Ultrasound of her abdomen was negative. I heard that Neurosurgery was thinking of taking her directly to the operating room from the CAT scan room. Don't know if she had anything else scanned. John, remind me in a few minutes to check the radiology PACS$^{\oplus}$ system to see what CAT scan requests were completed and if the radiologist has viewed them.

Dr. Louise: Where is she now?

Dr. Peter: In the operating room, I am presuming. She didn't come back here. Our trauma bay nurse is coming back with the stretcher but without the patient. Her head CAT scan is on the desk monitor screen. The amount of midline shift from the intracranial hematoma$^{\oplus}$ is remarkable.

Dr. Louise: Who is in the second trauma bay?

Dr. John: We expect that it is her seven-year-old daughter. She was found fifteen feet away from the

---

$^{\oplus}$ **PACS** – Picture Archiving and Communications System

$^{\oplus}$ **Intracranial hematoma** – blood collection within the substance of the brain

69

vehicle. Both her legs were fractured. She had a coma scale of 10 out of 15. She was transported with neck and spine immobilization and received supplemental oxygen. On arrival here she had a pulse of 120 and a systolic blood pressure of 80. It was decided to intubate her when she began to vomit. Her chest is clear. Her abdominal ultrasound assessment is negative. Her leg fractures have been temporarily splinted. Her pelvis is stable. Catheter shows clear urine. Her left clavicle is also broken. She has a good line in both forearm veins. She is headed to the CAT scan as soon as the intravenous lines are secured and Anaesthesia provides the airway maintenance instructions for the respiratory therapist. Her abdominal ultrasound is negative.

Dr. Louise: Any family members available?

Dr. Peter: None. One of the staff surgeons thinks he recognizes the mother and her child. The ward clerk is helping him hunt down office and home numbers. If this is the right family, the father should be returning home from a nephew's soccer game.

Dr. Louise: Any grandparents?

Dr. Peter: We are not even certain of the name yet. The police are searching the car compartments for registration papers. Edna, any paperwork found in mother's pockets?

Edna: No pockets; no papers. She remains registered as Female XT1 and the child as Female Child XT2.

15:25 Main Desk

Dr. Peter: The police just called. They have found a registration for the vehicle. The car belongs to a Matthew

70

St. John with a rural address some ten kilometres from the scene.

Edna: The surgeon has made contact with the husband and father of the patients. He and his brother are on their way to the hospital. Louise or Peter, will one of you be prepared to take the cell phone call from the husband?

Dr. Louise: I will take it, Peter. It looks like you have more than your share of paperwork to do. I will leave it to you to double check on the CAT scan completion status of the patient in the operating room. John, you should accompany the child to the CAT scan room with what is left of the trauma team. Call the senior pediatric resident to meet you there. I suggest you take airway intubation equipment with you in case the tube gets dislodged. You will want to monitor distal pulses in her ankles and feet.

Edna: Louise, here is the call you were expecting from the father.

15:30 Main Desk
James: I am James Knight. What can you tell me about the accident?

Dr. Louise: I am Dr. Louise and have just recently arrived here in the emergency department. First, let me know that you are not driving your vehicle.

James: My brother, Tom, took over the driving when we first got the call from the hospital.
Dr. Louise: Right now, all I can say is that we have about a thirty-year-old woman and a seven-year-old girl involved in a jeep rollover accident on County Road 7. Police reported a single vehicle roll over, just at the bottom of a hill. The adult woman has been taken to the

71

operating room by the neurosurgery team and the child is on her way to the CAT scan room. The police at the scene report that the car is registered to a Mr. Matthew St. John who lives in a nearby town. The police plan to go to that address from the scene.

James: That would be my father-in-law.

Dr. Louise: Mr. Knight, the police officer is shaking her head to the negative—the police plan to come to the hospital first. By the time you arrive we should have some more detailed information on the injuries sustained by your wife and child. The police will be able to fill in some more details about the accident.

James: My wife's name is Marian and my daughter's name is Janet. Was anyone else in the car?

Dr. Louise: I am being told, "No".

15:50 Main Desk
Dr. Louise: John, Janet's dad has arrived and has finished giving the registration clerk the demographic information. The trauma team leader has the details of Janet's CAT scans. She will be back after she checks in with the neurosurgeon in the operating room. Can you update Dad and me on Janet's status?

Dr. John: Hello, Mr. Knight. First, I will try to fill you in on what we know about your daughter, Janet. It is now more than 90 minutes since her arrival. Her vital signs have remained stable. We have sedated her and are protecting her airway with a tube in her windpipe, in case she vomits again. All the information I have about your daughter at this time is good news. On our initial view of the CAT scan cuts there is no evidence of serious injury

72

in the chest, abdomen and pelvis. The head CAT scan shows some bruising and bleeding around the left side of the brain, but no hematoma and no skull fracture and no brain displacement. Dr. Susan, the trauma team leader may have more details. She has gone to consult with the neurosurgeon in the operating room. The radiologist is looking at the various reconstructed CAT scan views of the neck, chest, abdomen and pelvis before providing a final report. It usually takes him about half an hour to go through a total body scan.

James: Can I see Janet?

Dr. Louise: Yes, of course, I will take you in. We just need to wait for the x-ray technician to take one last film of her left knee. We will explain the medications we are using, why she won't respond to you and how we are breathing for her. Edna can you check that there is blood typed and crossed for the child trauma victim.

James: You mean Janet!

Dr. Louise: Sorry, Dad, but we won't change the registration name until we have all of the components of the paper and electronic chart lined up. Edna will let you see her scratched up arms and face. Her collarbone is broken but that is not important. Janet's broken legs are swaddled together with a special wrap and will remain that way until she gets to the operating room.

15:55 Trauma Bay 2
Edna: Dad, come sit beside Janet. You can hold her hand but be careful of the IV line that loops around her thumb. Also, be careful of Janet's fuzzy brown bear. She was clutching it when I put in the first intravenous.

73

James: What bear? Janet doesn't have a bear!

Edna: Here, this is Janet's bear.

James: No! No! No! That is not Janet's bear. That is Luke's bear!

Edna: I don't know to whom you are referring.

James: Luke is Janet's little brother! Where is Luke? Where do you have Luke?

Edna: We only received Janet and her mother.

James: But this is Luke's bear. Luke would never part with his bear. He goes everywhere with that bear. Is Luke dead? Is Luke still at the accident scene?

15:58 Main Desk
Dr. Louise: Mr. Knight, we were told that there were just two victims. The police officer from the scene has just arrived. He can tell us more. We will ask him.

Edna: Officer, Mr. Knight is asking if there were any other passengers.

Police Officer: Mr. Knight, the accident scene was thoroughly searched for other passengers and for identifying information. Can we go into the family room? We need to ask you some questions.
James: I need to find Luke! Where is Luke?

16:00 Trauma Bay 2
Dr. John: Dad, your brother has your mother-in-law on his cell phone. He wants you to talk to her.

James: Give me the phone! Catherine, where is Luke?

Catherine: Luke is having a nap.

James: Bring Luke to the phone.

Catherine: But he is having a nap.

James: Now, Catherine! Do as I ask. Bring him to the phone. Now!

Catherine: Luke, Daddy is on the phone.

Luke: Daddy! Daddy! Janet stole my bear!

James: Luke, I have your bear. Uncle Tom is coming to get you and bring you to Daddy. Let me talk to Grandma, Luke.

Luke: Daddy, no want ice cream, want beary!

James: Yes dear, let Daddy talk to Grandma.

James: Catherine, there has been a terrible accident. Marian is in the operating room and Janet is on her way there. My brother, Tom, has offered to take my car and come to get you and Matthew and Luke. The car seat for Luke is in the trunk of my car.

Edna: Dad, come back to sit with Janet. When the orthopaedic surgeon returns from looking at the rest of the CAT scan images, he will explain what they plan to do about Janet's broken leg bones.

Dr. Peter: Louise, give me a chance to do a walk-around tour with John in each section. We will come back to review any handover details you need to know about the other patients in the department. We need to also review what the triage desk has been holding back for the last two hours.

Handover July 04, 16:00

Dr. Louise: Peter, are you up to date on the sad, sad story with the traumas yesterday?

Dr. Peter: Yes, Louise, I was told this morning that the mother was declared brain dead after midnight. The only good news was that there were no other significant injuries so a number of organs were salvaged for multiple transplant recipients. Janet, the little girl, had a minimal brain injury and two broken legs and a broken clavicle. She is in the recovery room after bilateral pin insertion to provide traction for her fractured femurs$^{\oplus}$.

Edna: Have they determined the cause of the accident?

Dr. Louise: Drunk driving!

Edna: No guff? That explains why the site police officers came here before going to the address of the car's registration? The police officer took John aside and wanted a blood sample for an alcohol level from the driver. I told the police officer that the patient was already in the operating room. He asked if we had taken a blood level for ethanol. John explained the formal procedure he could follow to get that answer.

$^{\oplus}$ **Femur** – upper leg bone

Dr. Louise: The family room encounter with the grandparents and the father was stressful for all. I will let John give you a summary as he sat through the gut wrenching details that came out.

Dr. John: Marian's parents knew that she had been to detox twice and had lost her driver's licence for driving while intoxicated. She had completed an in-house, four-week addiction program a month ago. Last week she saw her doctor about trying to get her driver's licence back. The husband had switched most of his work to a home base. There was little for Marian to do at home and she became restless claiming that she felt like she was in jail and would never get out on parole. The visit to the grandparents for half a day was meant to give Mom and Dad a much-needed break from each other.

Dr. Peter: How did she get the parents' Jeep?

Dr. John: She asked for it because she wanted to get the children some ice cream at the store in the next village. Catherine, her mother, inquired about her licence status and was told that the family doctor had taken care of that.

Dr. Peter: So, they gave her the keys?

Dr. John: Not really. As had been Marian's habit from her teen years, she had already fingered the Jeep keys hanging on the kitchen key peg. She had the keys in her hands before she announced the ice cream run. Then they discovered they had no car seat for Luke. They decided to wait until Luke took his nap. Grandmother was getting worried even before she got the unexpected call from Luke's uncle.

Dr. Peter: Why did the officer at the scene suspect drunk driving as a factor?

Dr. John: There was really no evident cause for the accident on a clear day with dry roads. The finding of the child so far away from the vehicle, and no evidence of braking in the tire tracks caused them to undertake a complete assessment of the surroundings. They found a brown bag with one intact bottle, half-empty, and another broken bottle of vodka under the driver's seat. The receipt from the local rural liquor store showed the date and time of purchase.

Dr. Peter: Do the children know they have lost their mother?

Dr. Louise: That will take some time to sink in. As Janet awakens, she will ask for her mother. She may or may not recall the accident. Luke has his bear but will be missing both his sister for a long time and his mother forever.

Dr. John: The phone call that James Knight first received from our emergency department must have terrorized him. At a later point, he was convinced from what he was hearing that his son was dead and abandoned in a field. The situation turned somewhat hopeful, but now he's hit with the demise of his wife and the mother of their children.

ENDNOTES
Chief Complaint – Multiple traumas
Vital Signs – 'critical' for two trauma patients; not known for the third.
Distractions: unidentified, multiple severe injuries, multiple victims, multiple caregivers

Snapshots of the vital history:

- The ultimate gift of organ donation will dramatically change the lives of a number of recipients.

- No apparent cause for a motor vehicle accident raises a warning flag.

- Ownership of a toy bear becomes a point of agony for the father.

- Power of addiction is constantly underestimated.

- The addiction risk permeates the life of each family member.

- Storage of a car seat probably saved a child's life.

What the father is hearing triples his agony. The question is paramount. The answer is needed now but rests elsewhere. The power of addiction strips a mother from her children and a daughter from her parents. Organs can be reused but time and decisions cannot be turned back. Luke's bear is returned to him.

7

Parents' Advice: Check the Records

Chief Complaint: Aplastic anaemia$^{\oplus}$
Emergency department team:
- Edward
- Dr. Peter
- Dr. John
- Medical records

Communication with:
- Brian (patient)
- James (father)

Handover August 01, 23:00

Edward: After completing handover, do you or John have time to talk to Brian and his father about some questions they have? His second transfusion unit of packed red cells is just about finished.

Dr. Peter: Yes, of course. John, please check and update us on the status of the two patients in section C waiting for Medicine to complete their consults. Check to see that they are in agreement that they will require inpatient admission for out of control sugars. Louise, let's go to the screen to make sure that you are aware of the status of each of the other patients in the department.

$^{\oplus}$ **Aplastic Anemia** – reduced number of blood cells (red, white and platelet) due to disease of bone marrow

23:20 Bedside Brian

Dr. Peter: James and Brian, Edward said you had some questions.

James: I've been reading about Brian's condition – 'aplastic anaemia' – and I'm wondering if the advice I gave him may have caused his problem.

Dr. Peter: I don't see how your advice could have caused Brian's 'aplastic anaemia'. What is on your mind?

James: Over the past year Brian has been getting 'strep throat'[⊕] frequently. He missed a lot of his high school classes; his mother and I worried that he would not be able to graduate. We were so pleased when he did manage to graduate in June. On his eighteenth birthday we agreed to reward him and paid for a trip to Cuba with his buddies. He phoned back one evening to say that he had another sore throat and a fever. I advised him to go to a pharmacy and pick up some antibiotics. Mom reminded me that we had done that on a previous visit when Brian's sister had an ear infection.

Dr. Peter: Seems like a logical thing to do.

James: He was better in two days. He was okay when he came home. Two weeks later he developed a fever and he was admitted because they discovered that he had a very low blood count. Then the bone marrow test revealed aplastic anaemia. Now he is receiving transfusions almost every week.

[⊕] **Strep Throat** – a common occurring throat infection caused by the streptococcus bacteria

Dr. John: Do you know the name of the antibiotic medication that he took in Cuba?

James: It is not a familiar name to me. Jake rarely finishes all of his antibiotic prescriptions because he gets diarrhea after a few days. We found the container and I wrote the name down.

Dr. John: I have never heard of that as an antibiotic for 'strep throat'.

Dr. Peter: John why don't you look it up? We occasionally used this medicine when I first started residency. It was a super antibiotic in its day and well tolerated. We rarely use it today. I believe that the only indications that remain are meningitis and possibly typhoid[⊗] fever. James, your concern is well placed. John and I will look up what is written about this medication's side effects and come back to you.

00:15 Bedside Brian
Dr. Peter: James and Brian, there is a long list of medications that are suspected to cause an idiosyncratic[⊕] reaction leading to the possible development of aplastic anaemia. Chloramphenicol[⊕] is one of them.

Brian: What does idiosyncratic mean?

[⊗]**Typhoid Fever** – a systemic infection caused the Salmonella Typhus bacteria
[⊕] **Idiosyncratic** – pertaining to or rationalizing that there is something peculiar and not understood about the interaction with specific individual(s)
[⊕] **Chloramphenicol** – useful broad-spectrum antibiotic available since 1949 for the treatment of a number of bacterial infections

82

Dr. Peter: It means that most often there is no specific reason known for that specific bad side effect. It just happens in some patients on some occasions, but we can't find any direct evidence of why it happens or why that patient was the target of the unwanted effect. For the vast majority of others, that drug has no noticeable bad effect. Sometimes there is a relationship to the dosage or length of time the drug is used.

James: So I was right, that antibiotic could have killed Brian's bone marrow.

Dr. Peter: Yes, it can kill the developing blood cells in the bone marrow. It is a rare side effect but probably reason enough not to use it as a front line antibiotic. The worldwide use of this antibiotic is still very high because of its low cost and long shelf life, both significant considerations.

Dr. John: In Brian's case, however, it probably was not the cause of his developing aplastic anaemia.

James: Why do you say that?

Dr. Peter: The most often cause for primary aplastic anaemia is never really identified. The clinical presentation of the disorder of aplastic anaemia often appears as continued unexplained bouts of repeated infections with or without fever and with or without easy bruising.

Dr. John: On that basis, we checked Brian's medical records over the past year. Before the end of May Brian had had four visits to the emergency department for 'strep throat'. An antibiotic was prescribed for each of those visits. Chloramphenicol was not used. On two visits, a blood count sample was taken (April 05 and May 20). The concern was that the repeated episodes of 'strep throat' were being mistaken for an underlying infectious mononucleosis.

Brian: Those monospot reports were negative for mononucleosis.

Dr. Peter: Yes, they were negative but when you review the actual cell counts for the white cells, red cells and platelets, each of the counts for those visit dates were far below normal. It would have been expected that, if anything, whether strep throat or mono, the counts for the white cells should have been very high in the face of an active clinical infection.

James: You mean that the disease was already showing itself?

Dr. Peter: Yes, that would be our conclusion. We just dictated a note to your haematologist[⊕] about your question and our discussion with you. We copied your family doctor and added it to your medical record. For you, the chloramphenicol medication was probably not the trigger for developing aplastic anaemia. Double check with your haematologist for her opinion, next time you have a scheduled visit.

00:30 Main Desk

Hematologist – specialist in blood disorders

Dr. John: Peter, does this mean that you will stop criticising the house staff for doing blood work for sore throats?

Dr. Peter: No John, not unless they are willing to interpret why they want the blood test, what they are looking for and what action they will take if they find the unexpected. On both occasions, there was an unexpected result, but it was ignored because it did not fit what was being sought. The accumulated visit histories in the medical records were not fully translated.

Dr. John: It is always easier to make a diagnosis when you know what you are looking for.

ENDNOTES
Confirmed Diagnosis – Aplastic Anaemia (eighteen-year-old male)
Distractions: life threatening diagnosis, repeated infections, parents' advice
Snapshots of the vital history:
• Parents search for a cause of their son's devastating disease.
• Available literature on antibiotic complications is easily accessed.
• Can scrutiny of past blood sample reports provide more definitive information?
• When should repeat visits for infections trigger a search for underlying factors?
• When and what blood work is appropriate for a chief complaint of "sore throat"?

The parents have raised a reasonable concern. A painful query is brought to the caregivers. The literature confirms the known historical relationship between an antibiotic and its propensity to permanently wipe out blood cell production. A more thorough assessment of the results of laboratory tests taken before exposure to the antibiotic suggests the origin of the disease predated this specific exposure to the antibiotic. The definitive answer was waiting for the right question to be asked.

8

Giant Butterfly: Listen to Mabel

Chief Complaint: Puncture wounds on hand
Emergency department team:
- Dr. Peter
- Dr. Louise
- Edna
- Dr. John
Communication with:
- Mabel (patient)
- James (father)

Handover August 23, 08:00

Dr. Peter: Louise, I have one patient from section D
to hand over. She is a twenty-year-old female with a six-
year history of inflammatory bowel disease. She arrived
after midnight with increasing anorexia, vomiting and
abdominal cramps for two days. Her pain has improved
with analgesia and IV fluids. She has just held down a few
sips of soup in the last hour. Her gastroenterologist
restarted her steroid regimen yesterday and will see her at
the beginning of next week. Admitted patients take up the
rest of the beds in D and most of the beds in section C.
Their admission orders are complete. The triage desk
wants to put a woman with post-partum bleeding in
section C because of a rapid pulse rate.

Dr. Louise: Edna, I would prefer Section A for the
post-partum bleed with a fast pulse rate. There should be
a bed in that section. On the screen, I see a child listed

with a puncture wound in A3. There is also one patient in A4 waiting for final serial cardiac enzymes. He could be moved out to the corridor.

Dr. Peter: Louise, come into A3 to see this young lady with John and me. Mabel is a three-year-old neighbour with the gift of the gab. Her father, James, is with her. John tells me that she has a peculiar "boo –boo" on the top of her wrist. John is suggesting that it is a horsefly bite.

Edna: Mabel, this is Dr. Louise. Dr. John wants Dr. Louise and Dr. Peter to look at your "boo-boo". I see that Dr. John has given you a squirt syringe. Dad looks ecstatic about that. Can we look under the pretty bandage? I will put it back. Does it hurt?

Mabel: Not now. Dad, can we go home?

James: In a minute, Mabel.

Dr. Louise: John, why did you think it was a horsefly bite?

Dr. John: Mabel was camping in a tent with Dad last night. She woke Dad up this morning crying about the hurting wrist.

Dr. Louise: Looks like two separate puncture wounds. Are there any other signs of mosquito or fly bites?

Dr. John: Not really, just some minor scrapes and bruises all over.

Mabel: Not squito! Butterfly!

Dr. Louise: Dad, what is Mabel saying?

James: Mabel keeps saying that it was a giant butterfly kiss.

Dr. Louise: Where was the butterfly Mabel?

Mabel: In tent!

Dr. John: Where did it go?

Mabel: Out door, to the moon.

Dr. Louise: How big was the butterfly?

Mabel: As big as Daddy's hand.

James: Doctor, don't pay any attention. She was probably dreaming. She was exhausted after a long day in the sun, fishing and rowing the boat. The butterflies have left for the season.

Dr. Louise: Yes, but where were you camping?

James: Just forty miles away, south of Highway 7, a small campground, just the two of us. This was Mabel's first overnight camping trip. Her allergies haven't allowed a camping trip before now.

Dr. Louise: John, what is big and brown and soars like a butterfly and sometimes bites?
Dr. John: Is this a riddle I am supposed to know the answer to?

Dr. Louise: Yes, John. You are training in a rabies-infested region of the country. Did they not even teach you about rabies at your medical school?

Dr. John: Yeah, but not from looking at puncture wounds.

Dr. Louise: The giant butterfly; the giant butterfly, John.

James: Oh my God, I never thought about it, Doctor. The caves next to the creek bank are full of bats. There are signs posted to stay away from them.

Mabel: What is bat?

Edna: Mabel, a bat is a flying mouse.

Mabel: Not mouse, giant butterfly!

Dr. Louise: Dad, the giant butterfly was probably a bat. Bats in our region carry the rabies virus. We will need to provide Mabel protection against rabies. I will call the family doctor and double check each and all of Mabel's known allergies plus her immunization record. We can also set up for the family doctor to follow up on the post exposure booster series and the final antibody titre level test.

Dr. Peter: John, let's see how much Mabel weighs and start the calculations for post exposure rabies immunization. Edna, can you explain to Mabel why you want to apply some special cream and special bandages to both buttocks and left deltoid.

Edna: Why three sites? Mabel only needs two injections today.

Dr. Peter: After John completes the calculations; you will find that the volume of the globulin$^{\circledR}$ is too much for a single injection in Mabel's little bum.

James: Mabel is used to needles from her allergy tests.

Dr. Louise: These are just the same but a bit more 'Ouchy' today.

Dr. Peter: Dad, let's sit down and we will explain why we need to give Mabel this extra protection if we suspect that she has had a bat bite. We will prepare a written dated schedule for a series of single injections over the course of about a month. Then we will arrange to measure her rabies antibody level.

Edna: Dr. John, what did you clean the wound with?

Dr. John: Saline and peroxide. I will repeat the same and put on a new bandage.

08:35 Main Desk
Dr. Peter: Thanks Louise, I should have made the connection. I was so taken up by Mabel's insistent expressions that I failed to translate her very logical explanation.

Dr. Louise: Just as well that Mabel associates her three needles today with me rather than you, Peter. She

---

$^{\circledR}$ **Globulin (Rabies Immune Globulin)** – used together with rabies vaccine to prevent infection caused by the rabies virus; works by providing the necessary antibodies until the patient can produce sufficient antibodies against the "also provided" rabies vaccine

might start a rumour campaign about the mean neighbour doctor who doesn't believe in butterflies. Let's complete the handover. It looks like a reunion from yesterday morning with the rest of the admitted patients in section A. Any transfers expected?

Dr. Peter: None. I reviewed that with the charge nurse about twenty minutes ago. The one new patient in A4 is waiting for his last serial enzymes. He is itching to get home. Says he will have nightmares about giant butterflies. Guess he could not help but listen.

Dr. Louise: Sometimes we fail to hear even when we try our best to listen. I wonder what made the father bring Mabel in for what looked to be such a minor thing.

Edna: He couldn't explain it away, and Mabel stuck to her guns.

ENDNOTES
Chief Complaint – Puncture wounds on wrist (three-year-old girl)

Vital Signs – normal

Distractions: insignificant findings, fairy tale explanation

Snapshots of the vital history:

• There are no findings to support the initial presumptive diagnosis.

• There is no reasonable explanation that the father or caregivers can determine.

• When uncertain, do we ask for another opinion?

• Can we translate what Mabel is telling us?

• What was the environment in which this happened?

Parents and caregivers have minimal experience with insect, reptile and mammalian bites. The child patient tries to explain but her words do not translate within the scope of neither the parent's nor the initial caregivers' lexicon. A new listener makes the obvious connection when the locale of the camping trip and the child's description of the attacker are given equal credence. Protective measures are severe but necessary given the new translation of the description that only the child can provide and vividly enunciate.

9

Bear Hug Tackle: Eyes Wide Open

Chief Complaint: Fractured ribs
Emergency department team:
- Dr. Peter
- Dr. Louise
- Dr. John
- Radiology consultant
- Pediatric resident
- Chemistry lab

Communication with:
- Brad (patient)
- James (father)

Handover September 15, 08:00
Dr. Peter: Good morning, Louise. John is just looking at a chest x-ray he ordered on Brad, the fourteen-year-old boy in D3. His father, James, brought him in an hour ago. I have not seen him yet but John has the details that he can share with us. There are two other patients from section D to hand over. The first is a sixteen-year-old with a past history of spontaneous lung collapse presenting with right-sided sharp chest pain. His oxygen saturation and vital signs are fine. There is a sixty-seven-year-old man with lung cancer who has come in coughing blood ten days after his lobectomy$^\oplus$ surgery. His vitals are stable.

$^\oplus$ **Lobectomy** – removal of a portion or segment of a lung

We decided to get a CAT scan pulmonary angiogram⊕ to rule out pulmonary embolism.

Dr. Louise: John, what can you tell us about Brad's problem?

Dr. John: Brad is a wide receiver on a junior football team for a district high school. During yesterday's afternoon game, Brad took a hand-off from his quarterback and ran directly into the opposing defensive back who stopped his further progress with a bear hug tackle. Brad was helped off the field complaining of right-sided chest pain. I suspect that he may have a fractured rib.

Dr. Louise: What brought him to the hospital?

Dr. John: Brad has been awake all night with sharp right-sided chest pain. He agreed to come to the emergency department this morning when he felt he couldn't go to school with the pain. His vital signs are stable but his resting pulse remains at 110. He has a tender right anterior chest, below the nipple line. There is no bruising and no evidence of an air leak. He cannot take a deep breath because of the severity of the pain. Brad has the body habitus of a rake rather than what you would expect for a football player. There is no back or abdominal tenderness. Shoulders and clavicles seem to be fine. Trachea⊕ is midline. There are no neurologic findings. Pulses in the upper extremities are equal. We are trying to get his pain under control before he goes home.

⊕ **Pulmonary angiogram** – x-ray assessment with dye injection to ascertain presence of pulmonary embolism or other vascular abnormality in the lungs
⊕ **Trachea** – main windpipe starting below the voice box and branching to right and left channels (main bronchi)

Dr. Louise: John, what do you see on x-ray? Peter mentioned that his father would like to see the films. Let's look at them first and then check with the radiologist.

Dr. John: You can clearly see the fractured right rib in the middle of the film. I think it is rib number eight. There is also some irregularity in the posterior right fifth rib. Can't see any pneumothorax$^{\oplus}$ or lung collapse.

08:25 Bedside Brad

Dr. Louise: Dad, I am the attending physician, Dr. Louise. Brad has one and possibly two broken ribs. He will need some pain medicine and we will keep him for a few hours to see if we can make him feel better. Were you at the game yesterday?

James: Yes, I saw the play. Brad ran off tackle inside the offensive end into the waiting arms of a middle defensive line backer.

Dr. Louise: Can you tell us about the contact he had with the ground?

James: There was no contact with the ground. The play was whistled dead because of no further progress. He never hit the ground. Brad dropped to his knees on the next play as soon as his offensive line went from the huddle up to their position at the line of scrimmage. That play was whistled and Brad was slowly escorted off the field.

Dr. Louise: Did he go back out?

$^{\oplus}$ **Pneumothorax** – escape of air into the chest cavity from a puncture or break in the lung air sacks or tubes.

James: No, the game was almost over.

Dr. Louise: Does Brad have any health problems?

James: Not really; a fractured wrist and a broken finger last year. He's been trying to put on weight but to no avail. He eats for three grown men. He is as skinny as a rail but really fast if he gets out into the open. Loves football. His coach usually uses him as a receiver rather than a running back. Two touchdowns and a hundred yards to the team's credit so far this year. This was their third game.

Dr. Louise: What happened last evening?

James: Brad did some homework, had supper, but even before he went to bed he said that it was killing him to take a breath.

Dr. Louise: Dad, we will be back. John, let's talk to Radiology.

08:40 Main Desk
Dr. John: What do you want to ask them?

Dr. Louise: There are three concerns. The first is that we don't want to miss a small pneumothorax. An occult pneumothorax could get worse once we assist the pain and Brad breathes deeper. Second, the mechanism of injury doesn't completely fit with fractured ribs from a fall. Finally, these fractures could be pathological fractures given his body habitus. Did you notice Brad's all-penetrating gaze? What do you think of a resting pulse of 110?

Dr. John: I attributed it to the pain he is having.

Dr. Louise: Let's recheck it after we control the pain. Could be the pain factor, but he has that omnipresent 'eyes wide open' stare. Most of us crunch our eyelids closed when we have severe pain. Let's get some thyroid studies and the radiologist's opinion.

11:45 Main Desk

Dr. John: Louise, good news and interesting blood results on Brad. The radiologist says no pneumothorax and no evidence of pathologic fractures in the ribs. Brad's pain is under control. His TSH$^{\oplus}$ is low and his T4$^{\oplus}$ is extremely elevated.

Dr. Louise: What is his pulse rate now?

Dr. John: Still 102. His wide-eyed stare remains very prominent. I have called the pediatric service. They will arrange workup and management plans for his hyperactive thyroid$^{\oplus}$ problem. I have already told Brad that he is finished for the rest of this football season.

Dr. Louise: Now you can also tell him that his days of being called 'a rake' may be numbered. Dad's vivid replay of the actual injury helped us to attribute the cause as more than a friendly 'bear hug'.

ENDNOTES

Chief Complaint – Query broken ribs (fourteen-year-old male)

Vital Signs – rapid pulse, painful respirations

Distractions: pain, body habitus, open-eyed grimacing

$^{\oplus}$ **T4, TSH** – lab measurement of thyroxin and thyroid stimulating hormone
$^{\oplus}$ **Hyperthyroidism** – Overactive thyroid gland producing a constellation of symptoms and some physical signs including susceptibility to bone fractures

Snapshots of the vital history:
- Coach's play call results in an unbalanced physical match up.
- Small body habitus puts an eager football player at a disadvantage.
- Detailed history identifies no contact with the ground.
- Are there any possible complications of this injury?
- What is the usual facial response for patients with sudden severe pain?
- Is there a unifying explanation for this patient's presentation?

Broken ribs can occur in contact sports when there is a violent localized impact. There is no such history in this presentation. There are no obvious complications. The vital signs, the unusual grimace, the small stature and the absence of a violent impact suggests that a further in depth investigation is required.

10

Assault: Speaking the Truth

Chief Complaint: Forearm fractures
Emergency department team:
- Dr. Peter
- Dr. Louise
- Edna
- Dr. John

Communication with:
- Steve (patient)
- Dr. James Smith

Handover October 03, I6:00

Dr. Peter: To finish off today's handover, B4 has a thirty-four-year-old female with a possible pneumonia. We will look at her x-ray and arrange follow up care. A fractured wrist is scheduled to come into B3 or B5. We are told that there are no inpatient beds. Neurosurgery is taking the eighty-year-old man with a subdural hematoma$^{\oplus}$ from A6 to the operating room. Triage has eight more patients. No known transfers expected.

Dr. Louise: What is the commotion in Section B?

Dr. Peter: The foul language you hear is from B4. Steve, a sixteen-year-old lad, has broken both bones of his right forearm.

$^{\oplus}$ **Subdural Hematoma** – blood collection on the surface of the brain and trapped within the skull bones

Dr. Louise: How did that happen?

Edna: Sorry to interrupt, a Dr. James Smith on extension 321 is insisting that he needs to talk to the doctor taking care of the boy with the broken arm.

Dr. Peter: Ask him to hold until we finish handover in a minute. The paramedics tell us that the boy has closed fractures of both bones of his right forearm. Splinted by paramedics; good distal pulses. Waiting for x-rays.

Dr. Louise: How did it happen?

Dr. John: He said that some big goon in the shopping mall parking lot came from behind him, grabbed his arm, and snapped it over the open door of his car.

Dr. Louise: John, can you continue to keep an eye on his distal pulses and his pain medication and see if you can get him to control his foul language. I will take the phone call.

Dr. John: That's where I will be. Are we sure that both forearm bones are broken? Are the x-rays completed?

Dr. Peter: Don't think so. The technicians are waiting to go into the room.

Dr. Louise: Hi, Dr. Smith, this is Dr. Louise. How can I help you?
Dr. James Smith: Are you the staff physician who is taking care of the boy who hurt his arm?

Dr. Louise: Yes, one of them. Why are you asking? Are you family?

Dr. James Smith: You need to know that he was breaking into my car.

Dr. Louise: Why are you telling me this? Do you want to come down and talk to the police who are here now?

Dr. James Smith: I would rather not.

Dr. Louise: Why not? Are you the person that broke this boy's arm?

Dr. James Smith: Someone else did.

Dr. Louise: Did you see it happen?

Dr. James Smith: No, but you don't understand.

Dr. Louise: Don't understand what?

Dr. James Smith: He can't have an assault charge against him. He is one of the star rugby players in this community and he would risk losing the American university athletic scholarship that has been offered to him. He needs to finish the season and academic year without problems.

Dr. Louise: Whom are you talking about?

Dr. James Smith: Can't say.
Dr. Louise: Are you talking about your son?

Dr. James Smith: Don't want to say. I wasn't there. Is his arm broken?

Dr. Louise: Dr. Smith, you know we can't give out patient information without consent. There should be a police officer still at the scene. Why don't you and your son talk to him or her?

Dr. James Smith: Maybe I should come down to see for myself.

Dr. Louise: I don't think that would serve any purpose. You would not be allowed to access any information on a patient that is not in your care. Get your son to talk to the officer at the scene.

Dr. James Smith: I am at the scene right now. I didn't see it happen. Can you tell me if charges are being laid?

Dr. Louise: Dr. Smith, respectfully, that is not my line of work.

Dr. James Smith: Even just charges being laid will result in his athletic scholarship going down the drain.

Dr. Louise: Let the police do their investigation. Get your son to talk to the police officer.

Dr. James Smith: You won't tell them about this phone call.

Dr. Louise: I don't expect to be asked about this phone call.

Handover October 04, 16:00
Dr. Peter: How did yesterday's handover lad fare with his broken arm? Was someone charged?

Dr. Louise: Well, yes and no and yes! The assailant turned out to be a senior high school rugby player who

103

claimed the lad was breaking into his car at the mall parking lot. The boy vehemently denied that when ambulance and police arrived.

Dr. Peter: What did the orthopods do with his arm?

Dr. Louise: They finally took him to the operating room late last night for reduction and internal fixation[⊕].

Dr. Peter: Was the rugby player charged?

Dr. Louise: Don't think so. The car belonged to the rugby player's father. The police found a metal bar with paint chips from the car door under the car. The story then changed to read that the injured lad thought he locked his keys in the car and because he was in a hurry to get to work, he had to break into his own car. He later explained that he must have made a mistake about the car.

Dr. Peter: How was it resolved?

Dr. Louise: Three important facts were added to the equation. The injured lad's car was a different colour, a different make, and at the opposite side of the lot. He had a suspended driver's licence for 'Driving While Intoxicated' and a few more metal bars were found in the trunk of his own car. The police wanted to take him to jail, but the trip to the operating room trumped that. Charges are pending for break and entry, and there is some question of driving with a suspended licence.

[⊕] **Reduction and internal fixation** – surgical operation to align broken bones and the use of internal screws, rods and bars to fix and maintain the alignment of the bone(s)

Dr. Peter: In assaults, we somehow never hear the complete truth first time around. Probably not even the second time around. Have you ever met Dr. James Smith?

Dr. Louise: Not that I can recall. It was a bit of an unsettling conversation. He wanted me to listen to him and for him. I have watched his son play rugby. I could not help wondering how and when a six-foot-two-star athlete might unload a helicopter parent.

ENDNOTES
Chief Complaint – Assault; broken arm bones (sixteen-year-old male)

Vital Signs – agitated

Distractions: pain, foul language, assault, changing details in history

Snapshots of the vital history:

- In the emergency department, patients and 'next of kin' may have their own agenda.

- Police often face similar listening challenges.

- Would colleagues try to circumvent formal communication channels?

- What are caregivers allowed to communicate to the police?

- Who is the assailant? / Who is the victim?

Screaming, swearing and conniving are difficult distractions to handle in the emergency department. There is rarely a good reason for any such behaviour. Not only the patient but also "next of kin' can exhibit unacceptable behaviour. Police face similar challenges in the listening process. The true facts need to be ascertained. The resultant injuries need to be repaired. Will behaviour improve?

11

You Don't Believe Me: Grandpa's Gift

Chief Complaint: Bowel obstruction
Emergency department team:
- Dr. Peter
- Dr. Louise
- Edna
- Dr. John

Communication with:
- Sean (patient)
- Mr. James (father)
- Surgical resident
- Operating room staff

Handover November 01, 14:00

Dr. Peter: Louise, the commotion you hear from C1 is from Sean, a ten-year-old boy sent to the general surgery service from the family physician clinic. He has a bowel obstruction and they are planning his operating room time.

Dr. Louise: A bowel obstruction in a ten-year-old is unusual!

Dr. Peter: Yes. He is a diabetic, but I am told that his sugars are good and his pancreatic amylase$^{\oplus}$ level is

---

$^{\oplus}$ **Pancreatic amylase** – digestive enzyme produced mainly by the pancreas

normal. His father, James, is with him. Apparently, his x-rays are quite impressive.

Dr. Louise: I have reviewed the handover list with John. Let me know if you have anything to add. Are there any expected transfers?

Dr. Peter: The trauma team is receiving the direct transfer of two patients from a motor vehicle collision on a remote country road. One patient has a severe head injury and the other patient is suspected to have a fractured neck. Not sure if both are coming by air.

Edna: Louise, the surgical resident is having trouble with Sean. He is scared and doesn't want an operation. He says that he just has cramps. The surgical resident took one look at his x-ray and is worried that his bowel will perforate if he is not taken to the operating room right away.

Dr. Louise: See what you can do to calm Sean down and I will come to see him. John, how do you interpret his x-rays?

Dr. John: Multiple loops of distended bowel with five to six small air fluid levels.

Dr. Louise: Small or large bowel?

Dr. John: Both.

Dr. Louise: Let's go talk to Sean and his father.

Edna: Sean, this is Dr. Louise.

Dr. Louise: Dr. John and I are the emergency doctors today. We saw your x-rays. The surgical resident tells us that your bowel is blocked off and that you need an operation to fix it. Let's see if we can get a better understanding of what is going on your tummy. Dr. John is going to listen to your belly and I'm going to ask your father some questions. Dad, when was Sean last well?

14:25 Bedside Sean

Mr. James: Last evening he was fine. He went out trick-or-treating and brought home lots of goodies. He had some candy and went to bed.

Sean: You didn't let me have any candy!

Mr. James: Actually, we had to take away his large loot bag. This was his first year of being a diabetic. He was really upset that we didn't trust him with it.

Dr. Louise: When did his trouble start?

Mr. James: He woke us up at 3 a.m. with stomach cramps. We thought it was from being tired and excited. He also had a two hour-long crying spell before he fell off to sleep.

Dr. Louise: Any vomiting?

Mr. James: No.

Dr. Louise: Any diarrhea?

Mr. James: Just a little watery stool before we left for the clinic.

Dr. Louise: Have his sugars been under control?

Mr. James: Yes. His insulin dosage has not changed in the last month. They checked his sugar when he arrived here.

Dr. Louise: John, what are you finding on your assessment?

Dr. John: World War II is occurring inside his abdomen. He has hyperactive bowel sounds, a distended abdomen throughout but no peritoneal signs on palpation. I haven't done a rectal exam but the surgery resident reported a cup of liquid brown stool. Just before I examined him he ran to the bathroom and released another bout of watery stool.

Dr. Louise: John, let's review Sean's vital signs and look up his initial blood work results. Sean, I think you may not need an operation right now but we need your help to figure out why your tummy is so upset with you.

Sean: I didn't do anything wrong.

Dr. Louise: Sean, I'm going to ask Edna to phone your mom to bring in the candy loot from last night and ask her to check for candy wrappers around the house. It may be that there was something bad about the candy.

Sean: I didn't eat that candy.

Mr. James: Are you sure?

Sean: Dad, you don't believe me!

14:45 Main Desk
Edna: Dad, Mom is on the phone for you.

109

14:50 Bedside Sean

Mr. James: Sean, you are lying. You did eat the candy. Mom found fifteen clear candy wrappers under your pillow.

Sean: That is Grandpa's candy. Grandpa gave them to me. They are 'no sugar' candies that he shared with me because he's a diabetic too. I keep them tied up in a sock so the baby can't find them.

Edna: The operating room is calling with a 3 p.m. time for surgery for Sean.

Dr. Louise: Tell them thanks, but the patient is not likely to need an operation. Keep them on the line and let me speak to the staff general surgeon. Sean, you will be fine but you will need to stay with us for most of today to make sure that your cramps and diarrhea settle down. You can expect to have some torpedo explosions in the toilet. We will arrange to give you some more intravenous fluids for a few hours. Dad, what is Sean's morning dose of insulin and did he get any this morning?

Mr. James: Sean knows his dose but I will double check with Mom. Sean hasn't had any insulin today.

Dr. Louise: Confirm the dose with Edna or John and we will work out an insulin maintenance regimen for today.

14:55 Main Desk

Mr. James: Sean, I can't believe that you lied to us.

Dr. Louise: Well, Dad, technically Sean did not lie. He did not have the candy you accused him of eating. Last evening was his first and most difficult unfairness of living as a juvenile diabetic. Later today, John or I will be back to explain to you and Sean how diabetic candy works to fool the brain. The bowel can't break down the giant sugar molecules. The large molecules suck in fluid from outside the bowel wall and the bowel becomes cranky because it is full of fluid. Cramps and crying leads to swallowing air which further distends the bowel. We owe you an apology, Sean; we should have listened to you more carefully.

Dr. John: Nothing made sense until everything made sense. Not unusual, but always a scary thought for us in the emergency department.

Handover: November 03, 08:00
Edna: Louise, before you begin your morning handover there is a message from the diabetic nurse educator. She would like to talk to you and John about participating with Sean to produce an educational video on 'candy for diabetics'.

Dr. Louise: John let's discuss this later. Your explanation to Sean and his father could form the basis for a short video for diabetics, family members and health care providers. Wonder if Grandpa could make a cameo appearance? Edna, I will call the diabetic nurse educator today.

ENDNOTES
Chief Complaint – Abdominal pain (ten-year-old boy)
Preoperative Diagnosis – Bowel obstruction

Distractions: pain, fear, planned operative intervention, impressive x-ray findings

Snapshots of the vital history:

- Caregivers are ready to act on important findings.
- Accusations of falsehoods bring further denials.
- Truth is rarely parsed through accusation.
- Features of the vital history do not align with the presumed diagnosis.
- An opportunity to prevent similar occurrences is offered.
- Reconsider the physical and x-ray findings in light of the recent diagnosis of diabetes.
- What are the criteria for an emergency surgical operation?
- Do we always seek an explanation of the potential causes when a diagnosis is made?

It is Halloween and Sean has pulled in a lot of candy loot. Why are you are taking it away from me? You don't trust me! You don't believe me! I did not have that candy! I don't want an operation! I want to go home! Can we step back as parents and caregivers to have a dialogue with instead of an interrogation of the patient? Are we too eager to propose final answers and solutions to what we interpret before we look at other possible explanations?

12

Stress Test: Call My Father

Chief Complaint: Chest pain
Emergency department team:
- Dr. Peter
- Dr. John
- Dr. Louise
- Edna

Communication with:
- Keith (patient)
- James (father)

Handover November 26, 18:00

Dr. Peter: Louise, in A3, there is a forty-year-old male, Keith, who was playing hockey and developed anterior chest pain and shortness of breath. Symptoms abated en route to hospital five minutes after paramedics gave him aspirin and two nitroglycerin sprays. His ECG and chest x-ray are normal. Cardiology has seen him but has not yet made the decision to admit. Cath Lab[⊕] personnel are still in house. A strong family history of vascular disease exists in both sets of grandparents. There have been no previous episodes of chest pain, no known hypertension and no lipid level assessments. No family members with type 1 or type 2 diabetes. John noted two other interesting facts in the history.

[⊕] **Cath Lab** – (Cardiac Catheter Laboratory) A special hospital unit where invasive assessment of heart function and necessary procedures are performed using catheters that gain access through extremity arteries and veins.

Dr. John: Today was the first time in twelve years that Keith had laced up his skates. Keith is also still on his final round of nicotine patches for smoking cessation.

Dr. Peter: That must be his father who is just going into the room.

Dr. Louise: Seems to be the wrong way around to have a father summoned to the emergency department for a son's heart symptoms.

Dr. Peter: Let's complete the handover details for the rest of the patients. Triage is good with only four patients waiting to be seen. Ophthalmology⊕ is waiting for a transfer of a patient with a probable penetrating injury of the eyeball.

Handover November 28, 18:00
Dr. Peter: Louise, how did Keith, the forty-year-old hockey player, fare the other day?

Dr. Louise: He did fine. He got admitted. His serial enzyme markers showed a slight elevation but his cardiogram did not change. They were planning to discharge him today but are rethinking whether they should do an angiogram⊕ given his father's presentation.

Dr. Peter: What happened with his father?
Dr. Louise: It was James, his father, who provided all the excitement just as both of you left. When the father received the call about his son, he rushed to the hospital,

---

⊕ **Ophthalmology** – Eye specialty
⊕ **Angiogram** – injection of dye into an artery to make the shape, contour and contents of the artery visible

had to park three blocks away, and then walk up the ramp to the emergency department. Ten minutes after he arrived at his son's bedside in A3, Edna, the emergency nurse, noticed that he was clutching his chest and sweating. The father initially denied having chest pain but when he was made to lie down on a nearby just-vacated stretcher, the cardiac monitor predicted the tombstone$^{\oplus}$ pattern on the anterior leads of his 12 lead ECG tracing. He had two bursts of what looked like ventricular tachycardia even before we started an intravenous line.

Dr. John: What did you do for him?

Dr. Louise: Oxygen, intravenous fluids, ASA, morphine, nitro spray, heparin$^{\oplus}$ and Cath Lab!

Edna: He went up to the Cath lab in a record time from symptom onset to needle. Eight minutes! That was also with the fact that the son was the one that the cardiology resident initially started wheeling up to the Cath Lab.

Dr. Louise: Same surname and same pathology but not the same emergency!

Dr. Peter: What were the findings?

$^{\oplus}$ **Tombstone findings** – the visual appearance of the electrocardiogram tracing just after the main upward deflection in patients experiencing sudden severe blockage of a coronary vessel

$^{\oplus}$ **Heparin** – injectable anticoagulant (blood thinner) used to treat and prevent blood clots in the veins, arteries, or lung

Dr. Louise: He had a clot removed and a stent placed in the proximal first inch of his left main coronary artery. No further symptoms and the ECGs today certainly show that the tombstones findings have been levelled.

Dr. Peter: That emergency department ramp elevated some thirty feet from the street, after three blocks of running, is certainly a great stress test for any adult. The chilly winds of a November evening added to the workout. The son must feel awful about Dad's cardiac event in response to his phone call.

Dr. John: Well, if you're going to have the big one, I can't think of a better set of circumstances and a better location. The son's unscheduled emergency department visit may have extended his father's life.

Dr. Louise: Certainly Edna's quick pick up and her immediate action obviated a catastrophe. With the coronary obstruction being so proximal, another minute of delay would have cost James a significant amount of heart muscle. Edna listened with her eyes and her head even though her ears heard that there was nothing wrong. Beyond the physical challenge of accessing the emergency department, the father had further demons gnawing at him. He had remarked, during Thanksgiving dinner, that his son was gaining a lot of weight. The daughter in law took over the discussion and Keith found himself signed up for gentleman's league hockey plus appointments with her dietician and his family doctor. On the first visit to the family doctor, Keith's blood pressure was normal. They tackled smoking cessation and a physical exercise program. Another appointment was scheduled to review lipid levels.

Edna: Keith's father also had a morbid fear of hospitals. He admitted that he had avoided doctors and hospitals like the plague. The last time he'd set foot in a hospital was when his son was born forty years ago, when he himself was twenty-one. Hospitals always made him extremely anxious since he was a child. Both his parents died in hospital before his teen years.

Dr. John: The cardiology resident confirmed that both paternal grandparents died in their fifties. The grandparents on the maternal side had similar young adult ischemic heart histories.

Dr. Louise: Great to have a Cath Lab. John, we should review the indications and management of thrombolysis for those occasions when the Cath Lab may not be available.

Dr. John: I have never needed to use intravenous clot busters for heart attacks.

Dr. Peter: That's a good reason for reviewing their indications and how they are administered. You don't want to be taking up time learning about it when your patient's heart muscle needs every second you can offer to break down the clot and reopen blood flow.

Dr. Louise: Hey Peter and John, did you notice that the son felt he had to listen to his wife, and the father knew he had to listen to Edna?

ENDNOTES
Chief Complaint – Resolved chest pain (forty-year-old male)
Vital Signs – normal

Distractions: father called as 'next of kin'

Snapshots of the vital history:

- Experience can guide caregivers to not accept an initial verbal response.

- 'Next of kin' and caregivers will some day become patients themselves.

- Is there an occult significant family history of this disease?

- Does the 'next of kin' harbour guilt, fear, or self-incrimination?

- Does the 'next of kin' practice avoidance of health care givers?

- When called, how would I best access my emergency department?

How will I respond if I am called to the emergency department? How will I get there? What unnecessary emotional baggage will I take with me? Will I feel responsible for something I said or did; for something I forgot to do? What are the risk factors in my personal health? What does my family history reveal?

13

No Nonsense Nurse: 'Double Double Latte'

Chief Complaint: Throat injury
Emergency department team:
- Edna
- Dr. Peter
- Dr. Louise
- Dr. John
- Anaesthesiology consultant
- Otolaryngology consultant

Communication with:
- Cynthia (patient)
- Mr. James (father)
- Operating room staff

Handover December 03, 16:00
Dr. Peter: Louise, let's wait for Edna to start the handover. She has just picked up a phone call.

16:03 Main Desk
Dr. Louise: Edna was there a problem with your phone call?

Edna: No, just very frustrating.
Dr. Peter: Want to tell us about it?

Edna: You know that we are not allowed to give advice on the phone.

Dr. Peter: Yes, I understand that it is a hospital policy in many places.

Edna: And the public is told that every time they call looking for answers as to "what they should do".

Dr. Louise: Some of the time they just want reassurance—someone to listen to their problem. Most of the time they want someone else to decide for them. Occasionally they are looking for a way to bypass triage and get to the front of the line.

Dr. Peter: How did you handle this call?

Edna: It was from a neighbour, a Mr. James, who knows that I work here. He got through the ward clerk by saying it was a personal call that needed my attention.

Dr. Peter: What was his problem?

Edna: His sixteen-year-old daughter, Cynthia, plays ringette on my daughter's team. Three hours ago she blocked a shot on net. The stick of the opposing player hit her in the throat just under her neck guard. She was breathless for ten seconds then seemed to be OK.

Dr. Peter: What is the problem now?

Edna: At home she has almost completely lost her voice and it hurts to say anything. There was a single speck of blood when she last coughed. A small bruise is developing in the front of her throat. He is asking me whether he should bring her in to be checked. Cynthia is refusing to come.

Dr. Peter: And what was your reply?

Edna: Peter, you know I can't give advice on the phone.

Dr. Peter: And what was your reply?

Edna: I gave him two options.

Dr. Peter: Which were?

Edna: Bring her in immediately!

Dr. John: And the second option?

Edna: If you're not here in ten minutes, there will be an ambulance at your door!

Dr. John: You would do that?

Edna: Do you have any better suggestions, John?

Dr. John: She doesn't sound as if she is in respiratory distress.

Dr. Louise: That is precisely why you want to see her now. If you wait until there are signs of respiratory distress, you have a major problem on your hands. The situation could worsen with almost any attempt you make to try to relieve the distress

16:18

Dr. Louise: John, Mr. James and his daughter are on their way to A2. Can you do the initial assessment as Peter and I finish the handover?

Dr. John: Sure!

16:23
Edna: Louise and Peter, John is asking for you in A2.

16:28 Bedside Cynthia
Dr. Louise: What are your findings, John?

Dr. John: Cynthia and Mr. James, Dr. Louise and Dr. Peter are the attending emergency physicians. Cynthia was hit in the front of the throat with the stick of an opposing player who was shooting at the net. She was short of breath for ten seconds but was able to skate off the ice. Over the past three hours, her voice has almost disappeared and she has coughed up a speck of blood on two occasions.

Dr. Louise: Any significant findings?

Dr. John: Cynthia prefers to sit upright. She has a tiny wheeze when she takes a deep breath in. She has a half-inch linear bruise across the right side of the voice box. Cynthia's father says there is a paper snapping sensation when you touch her anterior neck just below the bruise.

Dr. Louise: Cynthia, from what both your father and Dr. John have told us, we will want to start an intravenous line in your arm. Is pain or shortness of breath a problem for you now? I take from your head shaking that the answer is 'no'.
Dr. Peter: John and Edna, let's go to the desk to discuss the next step for Cynthia's care.

16:32 Main Desk

Dr. Peter: John, what are the available options?

Dr. John: Not sure.

Dr. Peter: What options do we have?

Dr. John: I am not sure I understand your question.

Dr. Peter: You look stymied. Let me offer some options for you:
- Ice pack, wait and see.
- Take a look down her throat with mirrors.
- Take a look down her throat with a laryngoscope⊕.
- Take a look down her throat with a nasopharyngoscope⊕.
- Intubate, paralyze, have a look down her throat.
- Paralyze, intubate, have a look down her throat.
- Sedate, have a look down her throat.

Dr. John: Peter, I really do not feel comfortable with any of these options.

Dr. Louise: Good answer. So what are you going to do?

Dr. John: Don't know?
Dr. Louise: Whom do you call when you don't know?

⊕ **Laryngoscope** – instrument to visualize the vocal cords and assist in removing foreign bodies and inserting endotracheal tube
⊕ **Nasopharyngoscope** – instrument to visualize the nose, pharynx and upper part of the larynx

Dr. John: You?

Dr. Louise: And if one of us is not here and you are the only attending physician?

Dr. John: Call for backup assistance?

Dr. Peter: Yes, John; Edna would express it a little more vividly and definitively. She would suggest that you invoke the 'double-double latte' approach for the bitter cup of coffee that Cynthia has handed to you.

Dr. John: What is that?

Edna: 'Latte' refers to your wanting to be smooth, soft and taking your time with your approach. To put it another way, you add aliquots of milk to ease the possible turmoil you may stir up. The first 'double' is that you need equipment for both a non-surgical access and view plus equipment for a surgical backup should the former approach result in near total airway blockage. The second 'double' is to find the two most experienced physicians to employ the coordinated approach to viewing Cynthia's upper airway.

Dr. Louise: We will call both Anaesthesia[⊕] and Otolaryngology[⊕] to receive the patient in the operating room where they have a second back up surgical approach to the airway ready if the airway becomes blocked or inaccessible to standard viewing.

[⊕] **Anaesthesia** – Specialty that supports airway, breathing, pain and consciousness

Otolaryngology – Ear, Nose, Throat specialty (also **Otorhinolaryngology)**

Dr. John: How do we explain this to Cynthia and her father?

Dr. Peter: I will do the calling from the desk. John, complete a double check on allergies, medications and past medical history, especially history of airway diseases such as asthma and experience with past general anaesthetics. Louise will come back in to explain all of the positive steps that Cynthia and her father have already made with Edna's directions. Then she will explain the plan of how best to continue to proceed in a safe and orderly controlled fashion. In the meantime, make sure that the difficult airway cart is always at Cynthia's bedside. Best not to display all of the equipment to Cynthia and Mr. James. No need to heighten their anxiety.

Edna: Already done! Airway cart is in place.

Dr. John: Any x-rays?

Dr. Peter: A portable chest and a lateral soft tissue view of the neck in the room since we have time. John, don't start seeing other new patients.

16:40 Bedside Cynthia

Dr. Louise: Cynthia, there is evidence that there is swelling, bruising and a possible tear on the inside of your airway around your voice box. You are fine now but there is no way of telling whether this will get worse or better over the next few hours. We need to look at the inside of your throat and voice box but we can only do that safely in the operating room. If there is swelling or a blood clot that blocks the airway, we need to get past that obstruction. If there is a tear of the lining of the airway, we need to see if it needs repairing and how best that repair can to be done. We are getting the team of specialists and equipment ready in the operating room. We will take two simple x-rays in preparation. You will not have to change your sitting position.

16:45 Main Desk

Dr. Peter: John, prepare yourself to join Edna for the trip to the operating room. We can expect them to call down to us within five to ten minutes. They are just cleaning and setting up the room. The anaesthetist and otolaryngologist are on site. Stay for the procedure if you wish. Record the step-by-step process so you can share it with all of us at handover tomorrow. You could design a future simulation exercise for your resident colleagues around this case presentation.

Handover December 04; 16:00

Dr. Peter: John, what were Cynthia's findings in the operating room yesterday?

Dr. John: First, they delivered a number of sprays of local anaesthesia in the nose and back of the mouth. Then, with Cynthia in a full upright sitting position, they inserted a flexible nasopharyngoscope through the nose. We all had a good direct look down past the vocal cords into the trachea[⊕]. They noted one small bruise above the right vocal cord. No clots and no mucosal tears identified. Cynthia remained in the post anaesthetic recovery room overnight and this morning she went to a step down unit next to Intensive Care.

Dr. Peter: In some patient presentations, especially rarely occurring life-threatening presentations, it is important to follow best practice protocols.

[⊕] **Trachea** – main windpipe starting below the voice box and branching to right and left channels (main bronchi)

Dr. John: Do the protocols all come with peculiar names such as 'double-double latte'?

Dr. Peter: Some actually do; it enhances their recall.

Dr. John: If we were to replay the history of this specific emergency department visit, Cynthia should have come to us directly from the ice rink. There is not a whole lot of room for blood or swelling between those two vocal cords.

ENDNOTES
Chief Complaint – Throat injury (sixteen-year-old female)

Vital Signs – normal

Distractions: normal vital signs, no significant respiratory distress

Snapshots of the vital history:

• Phone advice not available here.

• Listening sometimes requires immediate direction.

• Normal vital signs and a threatening vital history require action.

• Practised protocols help the care providers to keep one-step ahead.

• First, do no harm!

• How does one choose when presented with an array of uncertain options?

• The caregivers' challenge is to control the setting and obtain backup assistance.

Some histories cannot be debated. They demand that time is not wasted. Advice must be clear and unequivocal. Procedures that threaten life parameters need practice, experience and backup support. Clear explanations increase confidence and reduce anxiety.

14

Earth Team: Two Blessings

Chief Complaint: Arrest code
Emergency department team:
- Dr. Peter
- Father Jim (hospital chaplain)
- Edna
- Paramedic
- Dr. John
- Dr. Louise

Previous communication from:
- Grant (patient)

Handover December 04, 18:00

Dr. Peter: Welcome to the evening shift, Louise. John and I will stick around and give you handover after we receive the incoming code. Oh, Father Jim, don't leave yet; we may need your services. There may be a soul you need to handover.

Father Jim: 'Handover'? What do you mean?

Dr. Peter: If we (the earth team) fail to bring back life, you (the spirit team) may be able to intercept a soul fleeing from its mortal body and hand it over to the maker's judgement. We have a 'cardiac arrest code' coming in any minute now. How many souls did you save today, Father Jim?

Father Jim: How many lives did you keep from the maker's judgement today, smart-ass?

Dr. Peter: This is a young one. The paramedics have a thirty-year-old male coming in from a hotel in full code with CPR en route.

Edna: Any other information?

Dr. Peter: Not yet! Jim, why are you looking at me like that? Do you have somewhere else to be on a cold Sunday evening?

Father Jim: No but…but I am just worried about a former rural parishioner of mine, Grant, who is an alcoholic. I've been counselling him daily for the past three weeks. He was doing well, spent two weeks in detox and was waiting at a motel to be picked up by his family this weekend. The snowstorm yesterday delayed the family's arrival.

Dr. Peter: So what is the problem?

Father Jim: He called this afternoon sounding somewhat desperate. He said that he had not eaten for two days since a fellow detox acquaintance visited him, stole his wallet and disappeared.

Dr. Peter: From a drinker – a likely story. What did you do?

Father Jim: Well, I felt trapped as I listened to his plight. He finally agreed to my offer to send him a pizza from the shop across the street. He promised to come to see the hospital social worker or me in the morning if his family had still not arrived.

Dr. Peter: You've got to stop doing that, Father Jim. Feeding the hungry really isn't in your role description as a hospital chaplain. Why did he not come in to see the social worker yesterday?

Father Jim: He was too embarrassed, and he was hoping that his sister would come to fetch him this evening.

Dr. Peter: The paramedic crew is just arriving. They're still doing CPR. Father Jim, join us in A2. We will know what's up in a minute. John is in charge of the code. Speak to him about how you found this young man.

18:05 Resuscitation Room A2

Paramedic: EMS dispatch got the call from the motel registration clerk. He heard a commotion in the hallway. There was an open door to a room. The patient had fallen on his face half way into the hallway. Blood and vomit was scattered over the floor. On our arrival, patient was blue and unresponsive with no palpable pulse. 'No shock advised' on the automatic defibrillator. Oxygen was provided with assisted bag-mask ventilations and chest compressions were initiated. His colour improved. There have been some body movements en route. Repeat automatic defibrillator again advised 'no shock'. He is less cyanotic now than when we first started.

Dr. John: Continue chest compressions. Let's set up to intubate. Number eight endotracheal tube. I will take over the bag valve mask. Straight blade. Tonsil tip[⊕]

[⊕] **Tonsil tip suction** – the type of tip at the end of a suction apparatus; used to remove blood clots and foreign bodies from the throat

suction. What is the cardiac monitor reading? Hold compressions.

Dr. Peter: Slow, very slow rhythm with some funny looking beats.

Dr. John: Magill forceps$^{\oplus}$ please. Put them into my hand. Take the suction. Peter, a present for you. Return suction. Now, the tube. Through the cords; inflate the balloon! Carbon dioxide detector$^{\oplus}$! Bag tube ventilation at thirty per minute and then reduce back to twenty per minute. We need a portable chest. What is the monitor reading?

Dr. Louise: Regular rhythm at 120. Palpable femoral pulse is present.

Edna: Some respiratory efforts starting.

Dr. Peter: Father Jim is this Grant, your friend?

Father Jim: Yes, I think so.

Dr. Peter: Well to be sure, the Lord does not know what to do with you, Father Jim. The Almighty may not take kindly to his entrusted minister listening to the plea of hunger and then orchestrating the end of life of a faithful parishioner.

Edna: What does that mean? Why are you and John winking at each other?

$^{\oplus}$**Magill forceps** – angled forceps used to guide a tracheal tube into the trachea or a nasogastric tube into the esophagus under direct vision; also used to remove foreign bodies in the throat

$^{\oplus}$**Carbon Dioxide Detector** – measures the amount of carbon dioxide in the exhaled breath

Dr. Peter: Well Edna, John just took this out of Grant's throat. He had it wedged between his vocal cords.

Edna: What is that?

Dr. Peter: Two pieces of pepperoni sausage glued together with mozzarella cheese.

Dr. Louise: Father Jim, sit and put your head down. Take a few deep breaths yourself. Say a prayer of thanks if you want. Give us some time to go through our routine and then you can give your blessing and hand Grant back to us. Your trust was well placed. It looks like your friend Grant was really hungry. He was so happy to see that pizza you sent him that he gobbled it without chewing. He probably ate it real fast and then vomited. He somehow managed to get two pieces of pepperoni sausage to slide in between his vocal cords like a stopcock.

Father Jim: Will he be OK?

Dr. John: His vital signs look great and he is starting to move. We will keep him sedated until we assess his chest x-ray, cardiogram and initial blood gasses. Then we will decide about using a scope to look further down his windpipe.

18:22 Main Desk

Dr. Peter: Louise and John, let's complete the handover. Triage only has four patients waiting for stretchers. There is one stroke protocol patient returning from CAT scan and being seen by the stroke team.

Edna: Peter, John and Louise, come back to E2 for a second.

Dr. Peter: Sure, is everything OK?

Edna: Yes, yes, vital signs are stable. Grant is mainly breathing on his own now. He is starting to follow commands. We gave him some further sedation so he won't pull out the tube too early.

Dr. John: Why did you call us to the room? Why the whispering?

18:29 Outside Resuscitation Room 2

Edna: Look at the scene through the open door! Can we say that this patient is doubly blessed?

Dr. Peter: John and I thank you for your compliment.

Edna: No compliment intended, Peter. I was speaking of Father Jim's holy water mixed with his own tears as he is blessing the patient.

Dr. Louise: You don't see that picture every day. Thanks, Edna.

Edna: I am closing the door and kicking you out before you hurt Jim's feelings again. But the paramedics and John did a fine job, didn't they?

Dr. Peter: I meant to compliment the great teamwork. Poor excuse but I guess I was in a hurry to get out of here.

Edna: Admit it, Peter. It's always nice to have a special Father on your team.

Dr. Peter: How come they don't come to codes all the time like they used to?

Edna: Peter, don't get me started!

ENDNOTES
Chief Complaint – Code arrest (thirty-year-old male)
Vital Signs – absent
Distractions: no vital signs, young adult, possible alcohol abuse
Snapshots of the vital history:

- 'No Shock Advised' on two occasions.
- A pizza sometimes poses a danger for a hungry man.
- Jokes aside, practised protocols produce optimum results.
- Teamwork is needed at every level of caregiving.
- The 'final' handover awaits us.

Even charitable acts of personal giving can have consequences in patients who have problems with impulse control. There are many handovers in the chain of survival for the patient who has arrested vital life functions. With good teamwork the final handover can be delayed but not forever.

15

Space Masks: Family with the Flu

Chief Complaint: Influenza
Emergency department team:
- Edna
- Dr. Louise
- Dr. John
- Frank (security)
- Sharon (ward clerk)
- Respiratory technician

Communication with:
- Family members (mother, father and three children)

Handover December 23, 20:00

Edna: Louise, after handover there are three children from the James family in section D. They are travelling from Toronto. Ages: three, five and eight. Mom says they have "the flu". John is examining them now. No fever. Worst thing is their vomiting.

Dr. Louise: Thanks Edna, I will check with John.

20:15 Main Desk

Dr. John: Louise, I have examined the three children. The family is en route to Ottawa from Toronto for the Christmas holidays.

Dr. Louise: Why were they travelling so late in the day?

Dr. John: Dad got off work at noon and they decided to get out of town before the big storm hit. There was some blowing snow that slowed them down plus two pit stops for barf clean up detail. All three children have the flu with headache, lethargy and vomiting.

Dr. Louise: Any concerns on examination?

Dr. John: None really. I was going to let them rest for a few hours. Dad is going to get a hotel room for tonight and recalibrate the travelling plans for tomorrow morning. Mom is with them. She looks ready to start vomiting herself.

Dr. Louise: Is she pregnant?

Dr. John: She says, "No for sure!" She would not have tolerated the car ride if she were pregnant.

20:20 Main Desk
Edna: John and Louise. Mom is now vomiting. I managed to find another stretcher to get her lying down. Can I get her registered and give her something for her vomiting?

Dr. Louise: Yes, of course. I will be in to see the foursome in a few minutes. Let me first double check with Peter to see if he has any more handover messages.
20:30 Main Desk

Edna: You know, Louise, something doesn't check out here. My children have had the flu two years in a row. It's odd that these kids and mother all became sick at the same time. My experience is that one kid gets sick and as they get better the next one gets sick and so on until I end up in bed. Never had them all get sick at once. It would reduce the total grief time if they all got sick at once.

Dr. John: Maybe it was the car ride that brought out the symptoms at the same time.

Edna: Hadn't thought of that.

Dr. Louise: Dumb logic! Dumb, dumb logic. Of course it was the car ride. Edna, I am just going out to the ambulance bay to ask Frank at security about the car.

Dr. John: What is with the car, Louise?

20:33 Main Desk
Dr. Louise: Edna you are brilliant! Frank in security says that Dad was driving a really noisy late model station wagon. He directed him to the hotel down the street.

Edna: So what?

Dr. Louise: Edna, I will explain in a minute. Can you ask Sharon, the ward clerk, to call the hotel front desk and leave a message for Mr. James? Tell him not to worry but to leave his car and take a taxi back to the emergency department. He doesn't need a hotel room, since they will be staying in the department all night. John please page the respiratory technician. We need to find three children (ages three, five, eight) and two adult oxygen masks and set up connectors to get all of the family members connected to 100% oxygen. It may be easier if we use the

138

three beds in the corner with the two smallest sharing a stretcher with a parent.

Edna: Respiratory Technologist on the line!

Dr. Louise: Hi, a little unusual request. We need you to set up 100% oxygen for each of three children and two adults. Yes, probably carbon monoxide poisoning. OK, Edna; great question on your part. Let's call the lab and make sure which tubes we need to collect blood for carbon monoxide level.

Edna: Do we need samples on all the children?

Dr. Louise: Let's start with the oldest to show how brave she is and use some local anaesthetic cream. There is no rush. John, start explaining to the children about the space masks that mom and dad and they are going to get.

Dr. John: Do we need an IV line in the children?

Dr. Louise: Only if you can get the line without the need for a second needle puncture. Start dextrose and water to keep the vein open after a 100cc bolus for each.

Edna: Anything else we should be looking for?

Dr. Louise: No. Let's place the littlest on Mom's lap and the next one on Dad's lap.

Edna: Dad has just returned.

20:45 Section D
Dr. Louise: Mom and Dad, we suspect that you may all be suffering from carbon monoxide poisoning. We are going to start treating all of you. There is no risk to the

treatment and we will confirm your diagnosis with blood tests.

Mr. James: Why do you think that it's carbon monoxide?

Dr. Louise: Dad, I doubt that you have a Hollywood muffler on a ten-year-old station wagon.

Mr. James: No, the muffler just started sounding bad a few days ago. Meant to have it checked, but no time. Could you hear it from here?

Dr. Louise: Not quite but the car ride seemed to be a big factor in everyone getting sick at the same time. John, let's call the pediatric resident. Mom and Dad need an ECG and let's get that confirmatory negative urine test from Mom to prove she's not pregnant.

07:00 Section D
Dr. Louise: John, before the next handover, where are we at with the 'SPACE MASK' family in D section?

Dr. John: Everyone seems much better. Mom and the kids got a little sleep. Confirmed negative pregnancy test. ECGs are normal. The calculations for expected reduction of carbon monoxide levels have been made and all of them should be able to come off the 100% oxygen. We are repeating the measured blood levels on the adults and Pediatrics is deciding whether they want a repeat level for the kids. Everyone is hungry.

Edna: Grandmother is on her way from Ottawa with a van to pick them up later this morning. Their auto club will be contacted to get the station wagon to a muffler shop.

Dr. Louise: It is not every night that this section has five hissing space masks. There has been a constant parade of staff 'on-lookers' peeking around the corners

Dr. John: A big thanks is owed to Edna for questioning my diagnosis of 'triple flu'. She listened to the same history but her experience did not fit well with what she was hearing. Her doubt allowed a recalculation of the diagnostic possibilities.

Dr. Louise: This would be a case to consider for grand rounds.

Dr. John: Yes, the pediatric resident mentioned it.

Dr. Louise: John, you may be interested in setting it up as a game of 'jeopardy' with different categories of answers at different degrees of difficulty, breaking the group into teams with a revolving team captain for each question. Double jeopardy level could include the role of hyperbaric oxygen for unconsciousness, neurologic deficits, pregnancy and ischemic ECG changes. Let's also search for a final jeopardy question.

ENDNOTES
Presumptive Diagnosis – Influenza (family of five)
Vital Signs – Nothing remarkable, no fever
Distractions: Late evening, holiday time, number of individuals, ages

Snapshots of the vital history:
• Symptoms are identified.
• Patients are examined with respect to their histories.

- Presumptive diagnosis is made and accepted by the doctors.
- Something doesn't sit well with the attending nurse.
- Open team communication lines lead to a discerning question.
- When is the flu not the flu?

A virus is thought to disrupt a family's holiday travel plans. Everyone has symptoms. They can't carry on. A nurse is puzzled. She doesn't ask for an explanation but her uneasiness is recognized. The dots are connected. This family needs space masks before they continue on their journey.

16

Identity: A Suggestion

Chief Complaint: DOA$^{\oplus}$
Emergency department team:
- Dr. Peter
- Dr. Louise
- Dr. John
- Edward
- Police officer

Communication with:
- Mr. James (father)
- Phillip (son's friend)
- Mark (son)

Handover January 04, 08:00

Dr. Peter: Before completing handover, Edna and I want you to be aware that a police officer is using one of the interview rooms.

Dr. Louise: What's that about, Peter?

Dr. Peter: At 06:30, we received a call from ambulance dispatch saying that there had been a shooting fatality at a cottage about fifty miles away. On arrival the paramedics called to ask for a cease resuscitation order. No pulse; no breathing; no cardiac rhythm in a young male who had a rifle shot through his upper neck and

---

$^{\oplus}$ **DOA** – Dead On Arrival

lower face. The coroner[⊕] was called to the scene. A friend, who had joined other friends at the cottage the night before, discovered the body. Four young adults had planned to go deer hunting this morning. Police contacted the owners of the cottage. The mother was away for the weekend. The father, Mr. James, was home and received the news. The coroner decided to have the body brought to the morgue for the father to provide identification, instead of asking the father to come and witness the scene at his cottage. The dead body could be his son or one of his son's friends.

Dr. Louise: Does the father know his son could be dead?

Dr. John: Not sure. Edward, do you know?

Edward: The coroner is asking the police officer to have Dad identify whether this is his son, Mark, or one of his son's friends.

Dr. John: That is too gruesome a request. Could I suggest to the police officer that the identification could be done in stages?

Dr. Louise: What do you mean, John?

Dr. John: To ask a father to identify a son who has had his face exploded is unrealistic and unfair. I would first ask the father to provide any non-facial distinguishing marks and to show the police officer and one of us a recent picture. We could be the first line of identification to

---

⊕ **Coroner** – a government official (usually a qualified physician) who investigates, confirms and certifies the occurrence and the cause of death of an individual within a jurisdiction

prepare or remove the need for the father to look at half a face. Edward, could you ask the police officer if he would consider taking that course of action?

08:10 Main Desk

Edward: The officer said, "Absolutely yes." He has already been able to get Mr. James to list three specific distinguishing body features and has found a picture of his son on his cell phone.

Dr. Louise: Thanks, Edward. I will stay with Dad for a few minutes while the police officer and John go down to the morgue.

08:25 Interview Room

Dr. John: Mr. James, we took a good look at the young man's body. There is no two-inch scar on either thumb. There is no rose tattoo on his right or left shoulder. There are no earrings or earring holes. The right face does not have the appearance of your son's picture.

Dr. Louise: Who found him?

Police officer: I am told it was Phillip, one of the friends staying at the cottage.

Mr. James: Where is Phillip now?

Police Officer: Next-door cottage. He ran over there screaming in stocking feet and pyjamas. They called the ambulance and police through 911. They had been awakened because of the loud rifle shot. Phillip is now in the police car. I will see if we can talk to him on the police radio through dispatch.

Edward: It might be better and more private to have him use a cell phone; they can call our speakerphone in this private interview room.

08:31 Interview Room
Mr. James: Phillip, this is Mark's father. My understanding was that Mark, you, Allen and Anthony were all sleeping over and were going deer hunting in the morning.

Phillip: Yes, we were all here last night. Allen came late. I was already in bed.

Mr. James: What happened this morning, Phillip?

Phillip: Everybody, except me, got up before 6 a.m. to have breakfast. I told them that I had a bad cold and was going to stay in bed. About twenty minutes later I heard a loud shot that seemed awfully close. Couldn't get back to sleep, so I got up for some juice. When I looked across the kitchen counter, the common room was splattered with blood and a leg was sticking out behind the sofa. I thought that the guys were playing a trick on me. Last night I had mentioned that I don't like the sight of blood. This morning they made some remarks that I was having second thoughts about going hunting, and that I was just using 'the bad cold' as a way to cop out. When I looked closer, though, it hit me that this was no joke.

Mr. James: What made you think it was Mark?

Phillip: It looked like his socks; everything else was soaked in blood. That was where Mark was sitting all evening. I didn't have the courage of trying to look at what was left of his face. All I could do was to run out of there. Mr. James, the police officer wants to talk to you.

08:33

Police Officer: Mr. James, one of the officers with me at the scene has used the neighbour's snowmobile. He has caught up to Mark and Anthony. They say that Allen had told them that he would catch up with their snowmobile if they went straight north towards the edge of the lake, like they usually do. They had wondered about the rifle shot, but just thought it was some other hunter close to the gully beyond the access road.

Mr. James: Please let me hear Mark's voice.

Police Officer: My partner will connect you via his cell phone in a few minutes.

08:35

Mark: Hi, Dad, I am OK. Really. The police officer told me what happened with Allen. What are we going to do now?

Mr. James: First I will call your mother and your sister. Then I will offer to accompany the police officer to Allen's parents. Can you confirm that they still live at the same address as last year?

Mark: Yes, Dad, I am sorry for your anguish. Phillip, Anthony and I will come to Allen's parents' as soon as the police officers give us the OK.

Handover January 05, 08:00

Dr. Peter: Louise, yesterday's shooting victim had left a long suicide and farewell note in his bedroom at his parents' house. He knew that he wasn't expected home until late afternoon. They would have no reason to go into

147

his bedroom before then. There was absolutely no indication of how deeply depressed he had been, and how he fought to make everything he did bring meaning to his life. He was experienced with guns, but not obsessed with them.

Edward: John, Mr. James and the police officer wanted to once again thank you for your considerations about viewing the body.

ENDNOTES
Chief Complaint – DOA (unknown adult male)
Vital Signs – absent
Distractions: frightful history, uncertain details, police investigation
Snapshots of the vital history:

•   Expediency sometimes gets us too far ahead of ourselves.

•   Caregiver intervenes in the request for a family member to identify a mutilated body.

•   Team members can provide worthy suggestions to ease the emotional burden.

•   Although sometimes well hidden, suicide is never far from us.

•   Can you identify this dead body? Surely there is a better way to make identification.

Each suicide leaves many victims. None are prepared. Lives, families and friendships are annihilated into obscurity. We must strive to support each other. The stigma of telling others of our deep pain needs to be addressed. Dare to ask us to listen!

17

First Wings: Anonymous Gift

Chief Complaint: Recurrence of leukemia
Emergency department team:

- Dr. Louise
- Dr. Peter
- Edna
- Blood bank

Patient: Julia
Communication with:

- Anne (mother)
- James (potential donor)
- Haematology consultant

Handover February 13, 16:05

Dr. Peter: Louise, welcome to a relatively clean slate for Sunday afternoon. Sections A and C have ten admitted patient waiting for beds. Handover for B and D section involves mainly pneumonia and influenza today. There is an arm laceration and a twisted ankle just coming in from triage. John will be assessing those two patients. I'll be in the office for some time catching up on last week's mail.

Edna: Peter, remember our earlier conversation? Is it okay to have that individual come to speak to you?

Dr. Peter: Of course, Edna. I will be here for at least an hour.

16:30 Office Dr. Peter

James: Peter, I noticed your door was open. Do you have time for some advice?

Dr. Peter: Yes, James, if I can help. Close the door so we won't be disturbed. Edna has told me that she had a chat with you. She and your other nursing colleagues have noted that you seem distracted these past few shifts. Anything wrong? How are your wife and son?

James: Fine. OK. Everything is fine at home.

Dr. Peter: Is it work? Is something bothering you? Is someone bothering you? You look worried.

James: It's about a patient: Julia. Julia in C4 is coming to the department over the weekend to get transfusions.

Dr. Peter: Yes, I know her well. She's had some chemotherapy for her leukemia and now both her red cells and platelets are running dangerously low. Her haematologist has suggested that, instead of going home, she remains in the university residence for the weekend, and he arranged with us for Julia to receive some transfusions over two days. I discussed the timing with the charge nurse. Early Saturday and Sunday morning was the best choice for the elective but urgent transfusions. Is there a problem?

James: That's okay. No problem with the arrangements that were made. The blood bank has been very helpful. The written orders are very clear. Julia is using the transfusion time to get some course assignments completed.

Dr. Peter: Any problems with her intravenous access or transfusions?

James: No. It's just what she said yesterday! She was in remission for three months on two occasions, but the leukemia keeps coming back. Julia tells us that the haematologist wants to schedule her for a bone marrow transplant, but he has exhausted all sources for a suitable donor. It got me thinking; when I started nursing school, I was told that I had a rare blood type.

Dr. Peter: Sometimes it takes weeks and sometimes months before you can find a suitable match. I wouldn't be too concerned. Her haematologist didn't seem worried about finding a suitable donor when we discussed Julia's case. Do you think it would help if I talked to her?

James: No. You don't understand.

Dr. Peter: What don't I understand?

James: I want to be her donor. I was talking to Anne on the phone yesterday and I want to help Julia.

Dr. Peter: Who is Anne?

James: Anne is Julia's mom. She lives some seventy kilometres away. She is a military pilot. Last year I read an article about her return to Canada after fifteen years in Canadian air force bases in Europe.

Dr. Peter: Well, James, you and I don't have a lot of experience with finding rare blood type donors, but there's probably some volunteer organization in place that you can track down and arrange to volunteer your time with.

James: You don't understand!

Dr. Peter: Sorry, James. I don't get it. What is it that you are asking?

James: I want to be Julia's donor!

Dr. Peter: James, it's not that there have not been any donors coming forward for Julia. They have all been unsuitable matches.

James: I know that—I may be her only chance! Yesterday I had my blood typed. It is the same as Julia's.

Dr. Peter: What's up, James? There's something that does not equate. We do not go and check our own blood type whenever a patient needs a transfusion.

James: But this is different. I think we have the same DNA$^{\oplus}$.

Dr. Peter: Why? Do you know this patient? Are you related?

James: I think so!

Dr. Peter: What do you mean, you "think so"?
James: Long story. Long ago in a past life... I think we are related.

Dr. Peter: Get a grip, James. You've been working too hard. Beautiful girl, but get real. She and her family come

---

$^{\oplus}$ **DNA** – deoxyribonucleic acid; responsible for storing and transferring genetic information

from the other side of the pond, from Wales, as I recall, which I discovered when I teased Julia about her 'put on' accent.

James: It is possible.

Dr. Peter: What is possible?

James: She has no family match. Her father adopted her when she was four. Her mother and her brother are not matches.

Dr. Peter: How does that make you the match for the daughter? How would you have known her mother?

James: Almost twenty-one years ago, a young woman named Anne King was travelling to Montreal's Canadian Pacific Pilot Training College, having just finished flight school in Moose Jaw. I was on the same train.

Dr. Peter: Let's stop here. We need to look forward, not back. This is getting quite embroiled. I can understand why you think you should help, but aren't you are getting way ahead of yourself?

James: I have the same blood type.

Dr. Peter: James, you and I know that there are a number of immunologic matches that would need to be made beyond blood types.
James: Yes, and I want to do those tests, but I want to keep it anonymous. Don't want anyone to know.

Dr. Peter: Just whom are you talking about? Julia? Her family? Your family? Your colleagues?

James: No one is to know!

Dr. Peter: OK, James. I can see that you're adamant about protecting your privacy. I can check with Julia's haematologist about what testing needs to be done for a potential marrow donor.

James: Can I register as an anonymous patient, such as Mr. Smith?

Dr. Peter: I doubt it. Blood banks are very strict about their ability to trace back the sources of each unit of all their blood products. They handle their records in the strictest confidence.

James: I won't do it unless everything is anonymous.

Dr. Peter: Well James, simply put, beside the immunologic markers they would need to test each potential donor for HIV⊕, hepatitis, and all other transferable infectious diseases.

James: Will you ask?

Dr. Peter: If you want me to, I will talk to the haematologist tomorrow. Nothing lost in getting the immunologic tests done and doing the other necessary tests.

James: In confidence, for sure?

Dr. Peter: In confidence! No names used!

⊕ **HIV** – Human Immunodeficiency Virus; causes AIDS (Acquired Immune Deficiency Syndrome)

James: Thanks, Peter. My shift is over; I have provided handover for my patients. I've already said goodbye to Julia. Can I stay in your office for a few minutes? I need to clear my head about this.

Dr. Peter: Sure, James. It's not the best place to think, but on a late Sunday, it is reasonably quiet. I will just finish reading my mail and get out of here. Are you here tomorrow?

James: I have a day shift tomorrow finishing at 15:30.

Dr. Peter: Come by after your day shift, James and you can decide what next steps you can and want to make.

February 14, 15:50 Office Dr. Peter

Dr. Peter: Come in, James and close the door. I have just finished talking to the haematologist. He has explained what tests they would need. He actually mentioned that he got a heads up from the blood bank identifying that they had just reviewed a new sample that matched the blood type he had been searching for his patient. No names. Everything confidential. The haematologist just faxed me a sample requisition for the needed blood tests.

James: Thanks for your kindness.

Dr. Peter: I can fill out a requisition for you, and you can get the blood samples taken at the outpatient lab on the second floor. I will just mark it as 'blood test follow up'. Don't mention anything about a needle stick or exposure to body fluids. Those results go automatically to the infectious disease and occupational health offices. I will call you to discuss the next steps when I receive the results. Which is best, home or cell number?

James: Here is my cell number. Again much thanks, Peter.

February 17, 15:50 Office Dr. Peter
Dr. Peter: James, Peter calling. Can you talk freely?

James: Yes. I am finished my shift. Will come to your office if that is OK?

Dr. Peter: Fine, I will be here for the next half hour.

16:00
Dr. Peter: Hi, James. Come in and close the door. I talked to the haematologist without using names. Your results are back. The haematologist is willing to see you to ascertain your interest in being a bone marrow donor. He has a clinic tomorrow afternoon. You don't have to register for the clinic, but he would like to talk to you in private, at the end of the clinic. If you agree, I will give him your name and tell him that you will be at the clinic's waiting room area at 5 p.m. He wants to ascertain if you do have an interest in being a donor, give you a series of materials to read and set up a future meeting with you to discuss your questions after reading the material.

James: Would I remain anonymous?
Dr. Peter: Yes, the donor does not have to meet the recipient or recipient's family, but you have to understand two things. Your health chart will record the donor procedure. Secondly, the recipient and family will find it difficult not to be able to thank the donor directly.

James: When would it happen?

Dr. Peter: The timing would be the haematologist's call; it would depend on the response to the chemotherapy. Once the process of chemotherapy is started, marrow transplantation is no longer an optional procedure. The need for the transplant would be absolute. If all goes well, the time frame the haematologist is considering is two to three weeks of chemotherapy and isolation for Julia before the transplant procedure. The harvesting from the donor will require a few hours for the procedure. Sedation and analgesia is provided. It would mean no driving or work for one to two days.

James: That is a good time interval. I can take a few days off. Edna will cover my shifts without asking me to explain.

Dr. Peter: I can imagine that, like adoptions, the recipient can ask the haematologist to obtain permission to make contact with the donor years later.

James: No! No contact! Ever!

Dr. Peter: James, what is wrong here?

James: Don't ask, Peter. I thank you for your assistance and advice, but please leave it alone.

Handover January 10, 15:50
Dr. Peter: James, I need your advice on a communication sent to my office over the holidays.

James: OK, will you be there when I am finished in ten minutes?

Dr. Peter: I will wait for you in my office.

16:00 Office Dr. Peter

Dr. Peter: James, you remember last year when Julia, the leukemia patient, was in for transfusions?

James: Yes, very well. She got her marrow transplantation and I heard that she remains in remission at nine months. She graduates this spring.

Dr. Peter: James, I want you to know that I received a very nice letter of thanks from her mother along with a recent picture of Julia and a personal memento from the mother. I will let you read the letter.

Dear emergency department staff nurses,

Somehow Julia's visits to your department last February opened up her opportunities to get a successful marrow match. The transplant donor who wishes to remain anonymous has given a second life to Julia and returned her to our family in excellent health, as you can see by her recent picture.

We want to thank you from the bottom of our hearts for the kind and professional care you provided during the visits Julia had to your department. We know that these visits bought time for a courageous individual to be found and to be so generous as to provide Julia a bone marrow donation.

I have attached a small token of appreciation for your caring professional staff. Please accept my most cherished memento of my own professional career as an air force pilot. These wings are my first wings, just as Julia is my first child. These first wings have always represented for me a reach above and beyond our daily toils. Each time I look at them now, they remind me of the trials, tribulations and decisions you and I face in our day-to-day lives as we strive to go forward. Be assured that your kindness towards Julia and others who cross your flight path will never be forgotten.

As I continue to pilot the skies on giant wings, you will remain forever in my heart.

Anne King-Johnson, Julia's mother.

Dr. Peter: I have had this on my desk for a week now. My first thought was to put it in the staff room, but I wanted you to see it first.

James: Peter, thank you for that consideration. I also have never adequately thanked you for helping me with your advice and arrangements last year.

Dr. Peter: James, I can see the tears in your eyes. Why don't you take this home with you?

James: Can you keep it for me for a while? I have been very selfish. Julia's mother has figured it out. I have been such a fool. I have been unbelievably self-centred. I haven't accepted my responsibility.

Dr. Peter: It's OK to let the tears come.

James: Anne, Julia's mom, and I both came from adjacent rural communities in southern Alberta. She had been accepted to Flight School in Montreal and I had been accepted for Sociology at University of Toronto. For two days and two nights on the train, we spent every happy moment together. We promised to write each other. Just before Christmas, her letters stopped. No explanation. Just stopped. I never quite got over the hurt. I felt sorry for myself and have probably felt that way all of my greedy life. I never finished my program. It took ten more years before I tried again, this time, with nursing.

Dr. Peter: James, this worked out well for everyone. I would be honoured to keep this letter, the wings and the picture for as long as you ask. It strikes me that Julia's mom knew she was sending this to a special individual in her life. This letter, and these first wings will remind me of how fortunate we are to have you on our team. Come look at them any time; come claim them any time. Above all, ask me to listen, anytime.

ENDNOTES
Confirmed Diagnosis – Leukemia (twenty-year-old female)

Distractions: name of the next of kin, age of patient, incompatible donors, rare blood type

Snapshots of the vital history:

- How do we respond when a colleague ignores our common sense advice?

- What do we risk in giving an anonymous gift?

- Does a personal past disappointment shape all future personal interactions?

- Can we both want and not want to share personal information?

- Can we ignore the past forever?

A colleague asks for advice. A caregiver is convinced of kinship. Can you provide support to a colleague when you may not agree with the secretive approach that is demanded?

18

Finally Getting Stronger: Case Dismissed

Chief Complaint: Overdose
Emergency department team:
- Edna
- Dr. John
- Dr. Peter
- Dr. Louise

Communication with:
- Cassandra (patient)
- Mr. James (father)
- Cassandra's psychiatrist

Handover March 03, 15:00

Edna: Before you start handover, in A2 we just received, via ambulance, a nineteen-year-old female with a suspected overdose of acetaminophen. John is just coming from the room and can fill us in on the details. The father is out at the registration desk finishing the registration process.

Dr. John: I have asked Edna to draw blood levels for acetaminophen[⊕] and salicylates and get a urine sample for toxicology screen. I think we should initiate the 'N-

---

[⊕]**Acetaminophen** – pain and fever medication (also under brand names of 'tylenol' and 'paracetamol')

acetylcysteine'[⊕] protocol on this overdose patient. She looks really sick.

Dr. Peter: Tell us about the patient as we go to A2.

Dr. John: Cassandra James is a nineteen-year-old student in a fine arts program. Her father called the ambulance when he found her moribund in bed this afternoon.

Dr. Louise: Does she live with her family? When was she last well?

Dr. John: No, her father is a criminal lawyer who came into town today to defend his client in court. He called Cassandra last night and arranged to have an early dinner with her this evening before he returned home. The crown prosecutor failed to show up for the second agreed-to court date. The judge dismissed the proceedings and Mr. James was free for the afternoon. He knew that Cassandra did not have classes this afternoon. He had a key for her apartment. He arrived at about 2 p.m. and found her unconscious in bed.

Dr. Louise: Any pills around?

Dr. John: The paramedics found two containers but the labels have been scraped off. They recall that she has been here before, and her medical record shows three previous admissions for acetaminophen overdoses. The father is aware of those admissions.

[⊕]**N-acetylcystine** – used in the management of (acetaminophen) overdose

Dr. Peter: Louise, I will put in a call to the psychiatrist noted on her medical record.

Dr. Louise: Was there any warning of a decline in mood lately?

Dr. John: No! The father remarked that Cassandra had been looking forward to the dinner. She has had a rough time over the past two years. Lately, she has improved with respect to her depression. She is under the care of a psychiatrist who changed her antidepressant medications for the fourth time. She told Dad on the phone last night: "I am finally getting stronger every day."

15:00 Bedside Cassandra
Dr. Louise: John, what do you find on examination?

Dr. John: Completely incoherent young woman with pulse of 126, blood pressure of 96 over 70, dry mucus membranes and midpoint pupils that have sluggish responses to light. She is not protecting her airway.

Dr. Louise: What makes you concerned about acetaminophen overdose?

Dr. John: Her past history mainly.

Dr. Louise: You think she would try a fourth time when three attempts failed her? Did you do a cardiogram?

Dr. John: I think Edna was doing one as I left the room.

Dr. Louise: Edna, can we see the cardiogram? John, you look at it first. What do you see?

Dr. John: A fast rhythm at 122. Nothing else.

Dr. Louise: What else should you look for?

Dr. John: Not sure that I understand.

Dr. Louise: There are a number of factors that should alert us to considering a specific type of overdose in this patient. For Cassandra, the first is the rapid pulse. That finding is not very specific but it should be a trigger for further assessment. Note also the finding of dry mucous membranes and the sluggish pupils.

Edna: Are there any other clues as to what she may have taken?

Dr. Louise: In the history her father stated that Cassandra had noted that she was getting "stronger" every day. There is a higher incidence of successful suicide attempts in that interval of time when the patient begins to experience improvement. Cassandra's father emphasized her saying that she was "getting better every day" in last evening's phone communication. One more thing that her father said should be a concern to us: he mentioned that her psychiatrist changed her antidepressant medications for the fourth time. The likelihood that the psychiatrist selected a tricyclic[⊕] class of antidepressants is high. Now let's look at the cardiogram again. Let's measure the QRS[⊕] and QT[⊕] intervals.

[⊕]**Tricyclic medication** – drugs that block the reuptake of serotonin and norepinephrine neurotransmitters allowing more of these transmitters to be available for the brain

[⊕]**QRS, QT Intervals** – the measured time taken for the cardiogram tracing to traverse these specified predetermined points

15:25 Main Desk
Edna: Louise, the ward clerk has Cassandra's psychiatrist on the phone.

Dr. Louise: Thanks Edna, I will talk to her. Let's have the respiratory therapist set up for an intubation. We will need some extra help to initiate the 'Tricyclic Overdose Protocol' for Cassandra. Please add a tricyclic level to her blood work. I will come back to talk to her father in a few minutes.

15:29 Bedside Cassandra
Dr. Louise: Mr. James, I am Dr. Louise, the attending emergency physician. With what you have told the paramedics and our resident, Dr. John, we suspect that Cassandra has taken an overdose of her newest antidepressant medication. We have confirmed the type of medication from her doctor. Cassandra manifests the clinical features of an overdose of that medication. Her ECG shows evidence of the same. Now we have our work cut out for us. Your quick response will allow us to attempt to reverse the consequences of this wonderful but dangerous medication.

Dr. John: The ECG computerized report identifies the prolonged QRS and QT intervals.

Dr. Louise: This incoherent patient provides us a lot of clues to listen to, translate and act upon. The father's recollection of what she said to him last evening also needs to be put in context with her most difficult illness.

ENDNOTES
Chief Complaint – Query overdose of acetaminophen (nineteen-year-old female)

Vital Signs – critical findings

Distractions: repeat visits for overdose, critical findings, recently well

Snapshots of the vital history:

- Examination findings do not fit presumed overdose agent.
- ECG findings suggest a different overdose agent.
- Fourth change of antidepressants provides another clue.
- "Getting stronger every day" can point to increased risk of suicidal attempt.

Unlike a court appearance, after a suicide attempt, the case can never be completely dismissed. Everyday poses a risk. Every gain makes the patient stronger. Renewed energy raises the risk of the patient taking action. The dichotomy of hope and despair in mental illness cannot be forgotten. Historical and physical clues that will unmask the lethal agents need a diligent search.

19

Not to Be: A Father's Wish

Chief Complaint: Abdominal pain and vomiting
Emergency department team:
- Dr. Peter
- Dr. Louise
- Edna
- Dr. John
- Obstetrical resident

Communication with:
- Sylvia (patient)
- Mr. James (father)

Handover April 25, 08:00

Dr. Peter: Louise, the last patient John and I have to handover is Sylvia, a thirty-nine-year old woman with five days of nausea, vomiting and abdominal cramps. She's been trying to get pregnant, but she is quite certain that she is not pregnant. Her father has brought her to hospital but he does not know about her efforts to get pregnant.

Dr. Louise: What kind of efforts?

Dr. Peter: Sylvia is in a stable lesbian relationship. John, while I inform Louise, can you have Sylvia's father step out? We need to determine the actual details and dates of insemination attempts and the measures that were used to induce ovulation. We will also need to know if

167

and how she wants us to approach her father about this information. Her partner is at work today. Sylvia's vital signs are stable. Her examination reveals a nonsurgical abdomen with some mild tenderness in her left lower quadrant. I have ordered a two-litre bolus of normal saline and also an intravenous anti-emetic. Blood work and a urine pregnancy test are pending. We are waiting for results before considering the next steps.

08:30 Main Desk
Edna: The lab results for Sylvia are on the screen.

Dr. Louise: The pregnancy test is positive and her potassium level is a little low. John, are there any more significant details on your review of history?

Dr. John: Increasing nausea for the past three days. Sylvia has had some minor abdominal cramps and diarrhea, which she attributed to bad food. Her third artificial insemination was about four weeks ago, but there were no symptoms of pregnancy so she thought it of no use to follow up with her fertility doctor. On this occasion she was provided medication to stimulate ovulation. It should be recorded in her chart.

Edna: Peter, can you write an order for intravenous potassium for Sylvia?

Dr. Peter: Yes, Edna! John, has Sylvia discussed with her father the possibility of her being pregnant?

Dr. John: She had not mentioned anything to Dad about her efforts to become pregnant. She was going to, but had her feelings hurt when the screening question came forth at triage. Father had loudly grumbled, "Not very likely". Sylvia does understand her father's disappointment with the fact that he is an only child and Sylvia is an only child in a single parent family. He had hoped for a grandchild in the future but had stopped mentioning it after it became clear that his son-in-law was going to be woman. She is in there now telling her father about their attempts at artificial insemination.

Edna: That is Mr. James, the father, just stepping out. He said that he needs to go for a walk to clear his head.

Dr. John: Do you need to talk to him further?

Dr. Louise: Not now, John. What are the next steps in your plan for this patient?

Dr. John: Let's just see how she does with her intravenous and her antiemetic over the next few hours. We can get an ultrasound this week.

Dr. Louise: It may be wise to get an ultrasound today. It is unlikely that we are dealing with an ectopic pregnancy but Peter did report some tenderness in the left lower quadrant.

Dr. John: Anything else?

Dr. Louise: I would also get a quantitative HCG$^{\oplus}$ pregnancy hormone level when you repeat the electrolytes.
Dr. John: Why?

Dr. Louise: I am concerned of the age, the severe nausea, and the maintained systolic blood pressure of 150

$^{\oplus}$ **HCG** – human chorionic gonadotropin hormone produced by the placental cells following implantation of fertilized egg

with clinical evidence of fluid deficit. Separately each of these findings is not worrisome but together they spell out some possibilities that need to be eliminated from our differential diagnosis. Let's go talk to Sylvia and explain our next steps.

10:20 Bedside Sylvia

Dr. John: Sylvia, this is Dr. Louise, my attending for today. She has taken over from Dr. Peter who was on overnight. Dr. Peter and I have provided her all of the information about your history and examination. Your tests indicate that you are pregnant. If we can do an ultrasound today we would like to get that completed. We don't want to alarm you but we need to rule out a number of possible complications to this pregnancy.

Sylvia: What are you concerned about?

Dr. John: First we want to make sure that the pregnancy is located in the womb. This is probably not an issue but it needs to be ascertained for sure. We also want to make sure that you don't have multiple pregnancies. With ovulation stimulation drugs, that is quite possible.
Dr. Louise: We are also measuring the level of your pregnancy hormone. We want to make sure that the levels are not elevated and are in keeping with your dates.

Sylvia: Why?

Dr. John: Elevated levels could signal multiple pregnancies.

Dr. Louise: To add to what Dr. John has said, we also want to give consideration to the fact that an elevated pregnancy hormone level could also suggest a disorder of placental cell overgrowth. Do you want us to explain all of this to your father?

Sylvia: Let me talk to him first about what you just told me, and I will ask him if he has any further questions. This is all too much for me, and really much too much for Dad. It has been a long time since I have seen that weird but joyful grin on his face that emerged just now, when I told him about the positive pregnancy test. He does not want to talk about it, but I know that he still harbours the conviction in his mind that he did something wrong in raising me. He hasn't shaken the conviction that my choice of life-style was caused by a failure on his part. He keeps coming back to the same apologetic comment about raising me as a single parent.

Handover April 26, 08:00
Dr. Peter: Louise, what was the follow up to the thirty-nine-year-old pregnant patient?

Dr. Louise: Sylvia turned out to have a molar⊕ pregnancy.

Dr. Peter: How did Dad take the news?

Dr. Louise: Mr. James was devastated, but took it in stride. He was attentive to each word of explanation. He had apologized to his daughter about his off-handed remark at the triage desk. His last words to us were, "It was not to be!"

ENDNOTES

⊕ **Molar pregnancy** – abnormal form of pregnancy in which a non-viable fertilized egg implants and grows unrestrained as a mass

Chief Complaint – Vomiting (thirty-nine-year-old female)

Vital Signs – within normal range

Distractions: patient's father not aware of possible pregnancy

Snapshots of the vital history:

- An unexpected positive pregnancy test is a surprise for patient and caregivers.
- Sometimes 'next of kin' are not informed.
- When do normal vital signs need a more thorough critical appraisal?
- What factors make this pregnancy a higher risk for complications?
- What complications need to be ruled out in this pregnancy?
- What complications need to be ruled out today?

'Next of kin' sometimes presume to know that which they have no knowledge of. A patient's private life requires permission to explore and agreement to share with others including 'next of kin'. When vital signs are normal and the symptoms are significant, and the history is more complex, there is a possibility that there is more than a single simple explanation for the patient's condition.

20

Too Much Milk: Yes I Can

Chief Complaint: Rash
Emergency department team:
- Dr. Peter
- Dr. Louise
- Dr. John
- Edna

Communication with:
- Mr. James (father)
- Donna (patient)

Handover May 27, 16:00

Dr. Peter: Louise, I have written down the names, location, responsible service attachment and diagnoses for the admitted patients remaining in the department. There are two more patients in section A waiting for their last serial heart enzymes levels. They have their discharge and follow-up appointments arranged. Triage has eight patients. In B4 we have Donna, a six-year-old girl whom I have not seen yet. Edna says Donna has tiny bluish pinpoint spots on her lower legs. John has just assessed her. John, have you completed the workup, or do we need to handover the care for Donna?

Dr. John: I am not sure how far we should investigate. Donna and her father, James, were at the walk-in clinic, and they were sent here for tests. Each spot is about two to three millimetres in size and there are seven to nine in each lower leg below the knees. There are three fading spots on her left forearm. They actually look like mosquito bites, but there is some bluish discoloration.

Dr. Louise: Is there any significant history?

Dr. John: There has been no fever, no known contact with infectious diseases and no stomach upsets or diarrhea. There is no other bruising or skin discoloration.

Dr. Louise: How long have the blue spots been there?

Dr. John: According to her father, at least four to five days. Their pattern changes and sometimes they are more noticeable than at other times.

Dr. Louise: Are they itchy?

Dr. John: Occasionally, especially at night.

Dr. Louise: Any new foods?

Dr. John: No, but the father wonders if it's the milk.

Dr. Louise: Why?

Dr. John: Donna seems to be drinking a lot more milk every day.

Dr. Louise: John, what do you find on the rest of the examination?

Dr. John: Ears, throat and neck are normal. Chest and abdominal examinations are normal. No swollen lymph glands. Each spot is a little raised and some spots seem to have a central indentation.

Dr. Louise: What do you want to do, John?

Dr. John: I would like you to look at the lesions. It is reasonable to do a platelet count. There is nothing to suggest infection or a 'vasculitis'[⊕]. Donna is thinking about giving us a urine sample.

16:10 Bedside Donna
Dr. Louise: Let's ask Dad some more questions. Mr. James, I am Dr. Louise. Dr. John has told me about Donna's spots. Do you have any animals around the house?

Mr. James: No, our house is very clean. Donna has been asking for a kitten, but she is too young to take care of a cat.

Donna: Yes I can! I am not too little!

Dr. Louise: Donna, I am Dr. Louise. Do any of your friends have cats or dogs?

Donna: My cousin Maria is eight years old and she has a cat.

Mr. James: Dr. Louise, Maria lives on a farm, two hundred kilometres from us.

Dr. Louise: Donna, what do kittens like to eat?

Donna: Milk and fish!

[⊕] **Vasculitis** – a group of disorders affecting a variety of organs; caused by infection or inflammation of specific blood vessels

Dr. Louise: What else do kittens need?

Donna: They are very clean. Maria says they need love and litter and a quiet room to rest!

Dr. Louise: Dad, could you go out to the desk and ask the ward clerk to direct you to the water fountain to get Donna a drink of water? We are waiting for a urine sample from her. Take your time in returning; Donna, John and I are going to have a little chat so she can tell us what she knows about taking care of kittens. We will come out and get you.

16:20
Dr. Louise: Donna, Dr. John wants to know your kitten's name?

Donna: Rufus.

Dr. Louise: Where does he sleep?

Donna: He has a bed in the tool shed. I bring him milk every morning and after school. He eats all the fish that I don't like. The dogs and cats in the neighbourhood are really mean. Rufus is scared of them. If I had a cat cage, I could take Rufus to school. He likes to curl up in a ball on my lap or between my feet while I do my spelling homework.

16:25
Dr. Louise: Mr. James, come back in. We have found the missing piece to the puzzle. Donna has adopted a stray neighbourhood kitten. I have asked her to tell you how well she has been taking care of Rufus, her adopted kitten, and how she is protecting it from mean neighbourhood

cats and dogs. Donna has been sharing her extra milk with Rufus.

Mr. James: Are you saying these are fleabites?

Dr. Louise: Yes! The fleabites are nothing to worry about but if you decide to bring the kitten inside, you may want to visit the vet for some kind of a spray or drop medication. Mr. James, you have an outstanding daughter. It was a pleasure for John and I to listen to Donna.

ENDNOTES
Chief Complaint – Rash on lower legs (seven-year-old girl)

Vital Signs – normal

Distractions: referred, unexplained rash, too little, too much milk, yes I can

Snapshots of the vital history:
- Location and appearance of rash.
- Healthy child.
- Confident child.
- Willing historian of her capabilities.
- Let the child speak of what she knows!

Children are cute. Children are determined. Children are ingenious. Children are straight arrows with their health care providers when approached in a positive frame of conversation. What more could a parent ask from their child's visit to the emergency department. Worse fears on arrival can turn into wide smiles on departure.

21

Pain in the Neck: Missed X-Ray Finding

Chief Complaint: Pain in the neck
Emergency department team:
- Dr. Peter
- Dr. Louise
- Dr. John
- Edna
- Ward clerk
Communication with:
- Gilbert (patient)
- Mr. James (father)
- Randy (brother)

Handover August 13, 08:10
Dr. Peter: Louise, welcome to the beginning of the dayshift. The night was kind to us. When we are through handover, I also have a missed x-ray finding to follow up.

Dr. Louise: Was it one of mine?

Dr. Peter: No, it is one of my patients. Gilbert James is a twenty-five-year old male with a sore neck. John and I saw him, late in the evening, a few days ago. We didn't recognize an abnormality on the x-ray; we didn't think that the mechanism of injury warranted any further imaging at the time. The radiologist reports an undisplaced but potentially unstable fracture of the second vertebrae[⊕]. The radiologist is asking for a CAT scan.

Dr. Louise: How did it happen?

Dr. John: He said he was trying to get into his car via the trunk hatchback door. He needed to pull out his musical instruments without scratching the car that was parked immediately beside his car. He climbed in but all of a sudden slipped forward hitting his head against the front dashboard. He was OK at the time, but when he woke up the next morning, he had a constant pain down the back of his neck. On examination, he had tenderness over the back of the neck, and a reduced range of movement. There were no other findings.

Dr. Peter: I reviewed the x-rays with John, and I thought they were normal. Now I need to contact Gilbert. Oh great, he has an 'out of town' address. This is not going to be easy. No one seems to be answering his phone. Maybe it is not the correct number.

Edna: Let's ask the ward clerk to look up his last name in the phone listing. There can't be too many entries with the same last name in such a small town.

Ward Clerk: I have ten listings with the same last name. Where do you want me to start?
Edna: Next of kin is recorded as Mary, his mother.

Ward Clerk: Mary, not listed; not even a Joseph.

Dr. John: Could we try the family physician's office?

[⊕]**Vertebrae** – bony blocks that make up the skeletal framework that protects the spinal cord

Dr. Peter: There is no family doctor recorded on his chart.

Edna: There is only one doctor's office in that town. Someone in that office may know the names of Gilbert's next of kin.

08:35
Ward Clerk: Got his father's name and number from the secretary at the family doctor's office. David, do you want to connect?

Dr. Peter: Yes, please. Louise, there are no further patients to hand over. I will make this phone call and then update you.

Dr. John: I hope someone is at home. The more I look at this x-ray, the more I feel the urgency to put a collar on Gilbert's neck.

Dr. Peter: Mr. James, I am Dr. Peter from the Regional General Hospital emergency department. We need to get in contact with your son, Gilbert. We saw him two days ago with a sore neck, and our radiologist wants to take more x-rays.

Mr. James: He told me about it. He still has a very sore neck.

Dr. Peter: Is he there? Can I talk to him?
Mr. James: No, he is actually driving to your city as we speak. He left two heavy pieces of equipment at the high school auditorium. He's picking them up en route to another 'gig' his band is playing tonight in a neighbouring school.

Dr. Peter: Do you know the name of the school where he left his equipment?

Mr. James: No, but his little brother was there last weekend. I will have him call you when he gets out of the shower.

Dr. Peter: Yes, please! It is extremely important. The ward clerk will give you our direct phone number.

08:45
Ward Clerk: Peter, we are catching up to Gilbert. His brother called back. Gilbert will be at St. Laurent Secondary School within the next hour to pick up his music equipment. I know the custodian there and have called him. He will be on the lookout for a gimpy musician. The caretaker has the keys to the room where the instruments are stored. He has the number for the direct line to my desk.

09:10
Edna: Peter, you have a phone call from Gilbert, 'the pain in the neck' patient. Line 647.

Gilbert: Hi, Doctor, I was going to drop in today. The pain in my neck is so bad that I don't think I can play tonight.

Dr. Peter: It is important that you get here right away. The radiologist wants to make sure that you don't have a fracture high up in your neck. It is important that you don't bend or twist your head.

Gilbert: It hurts too much! The custodian at the school has kindly offered to drive me to the hospital.

Dr. Peter: Please don't try moving any more equipment or instruments into or out of your car. I just don't understand how you could have injured your cervical vertebrae with a small slip inside your hatchback car.

Gilbert: Well, I had better come clean on that one. I did not hurt it in the car.

Dr. Peter: How did you hurt your neck?

Gilbert: It definitely occurred later in the evening. I fell backwards trying to do a headstand. I didn't want the nurses and doctors listening to my story to not take me seriously, so I made up the story of the slip-and-fall inside the car. The car situation actually happened to me two years ago.

Dr. Peter: Gilbert, we will take you seriously. A collar will be waiting for you at the triage desk. Dr. John, our resident, remembers you, and today's staff physician, Dr. Louise, will coordinate your CAT scan. They will get any necessary consultations. Did you have any x-rays two years ago?

Gilbert: No, everything resolved in three days.

Dr. Louise: Scary thought! A young man is walking around with a possible broken neck. It is hard to be sceptical when one is listening to an explanation of how it happened.

Dr. John: After today, my scepticism monitor will need to be recalibrated!

ENDNOTES

Chief Complaint – Sore neck (twenty-five-year-old male)

Vital Signs – normal

Distractions: no serious mechanism of injury

Snapshots of the vital history:

- Patients want to be taken seriously.
- Altered history affects the diagnostic mind set.
- Sometimes we need to track down 'next of kin'.
- In hindsight, a suboptimal interpretation of requested x-rays is difficult to defend.

Do patients colour their history so they will not look foolish? First person communication without corroboration can be incomplete or just false when it addresses unusual injury. An accompanying next of kin or friend may have painted a different lens for this camera. A detailed history of the mechanism of injury is very relevant in determining the need for x-rays of the neck. Mechanism of injury does not change the need to accurately interpret the requested x-ray.

22

No One Asked: Truth or Consequence

Chief Complaint: Blood in urine
Emergency department team:
- Dr. Peter
- Dr. John
- Dr. Louise
- Edna
Communication with:
- Leonard (patient)
- James (father)

Handover May 29, 16:00
Dr. Peter: Louise, I don't have any further patients to handover. Triage has six patients waiting to be seen. There are no expected transfers or ambulance arrivals. John, tell Louise about the patient we have in B4.

Dr. John: Leonard, in B4, is a fifteen-year-old male with gross blood in his urine. His eighteen-year-old sister came home for lunch, and she noticed the blood in the toilet bowl. After questioning him, she took charge and brought him to the emergency department. We are waiting for his father to come in to sign consent for a contrast intravenous study of his kidneys and a cystoscopy[⊕].

⊕ **Cystoscopy** – visual examination of the inside of the urinary bladder with a special instrument

Dr. Louise: Fill us in on the history.

Dr. John: Leonard James is a shy, grade nine student who stayed home from classes today nursing a sprained ankle he received playing soccer two days ago. He was resting in bed until he got up to go urinate. He noted bright red blood in his urine. It has never happened before. There was no pain.

Dr. Louise: Any medications?

Dr. John: No.

Dr. Louise: Any trauma, assaults, falls, back injury?

Dr. John: No history of injury. His vital signs are normal. Examinations of his back, abdomen, groins, scrotum and penis are normal except for a drop of blood at the opening of his urethra⊕. Ultrasound of his abdomen is normal.

Dr. Louise: Why do you want to do an intravenous x-ray study?

Dr. John: To rule out a vascular abnormality or cyst or kidney trauma.

Dr. Louise: Ultrasound is diagnostic for most of those concerns. What will you do if the intravenous dye study is normal?

Dr. John: We have already talked to the Urology⊕ Service to arrange a cystoscopy.

⊕ **Urethra** – drainage channel from bladder exiting at external genitalia

⊕ **Urology** – Specialty for disorders of urinary system

Dr. Louise: What does the urine show here now, after three hours?

Dr. John: Amazingly clear with two small one-half centimetre clots. Microscopy shows red blood cells with no evidence of casts or crystals.

Dr. Louise: Any other findings with the rest of the physical exam?

Dr. John: Completely normal! There is some mild swelling on the side of the right foot...getting better according to Leonard.

16:35
Dr. Louise: Edna, is this Leonard's dad?

Edna: Yes, Mr. James is Leonard's dad. This is Dr. Louise, the attending emergency physician.

Dr. Louise: Hello, Mr. James. You don't remember me but I was a student in your chemistry class many years ago. I am the attending physician who has just taken over from Dr. Peter. Dr. John is our emergency medicine resident. They called you because we need you to sign permission for an intravenous dye contrast study. As you know, your daughter brought Leonard to our emergency department shortly after the noon hour because there was blood in his urine. Nothing serious was found on examination but the thinking was that this unusual occurrence should be investigated.

Dr. John: Dr. Louise, Edna is telling us that Leonard is refusing to have the investigations. I am scheduled to go to a seminar starting at 16:30.

Dr. Louise: Thanks, John, go ahead. Dad, I haven't seen Leonard yet but, from what I am hearing, I suggest that you take the opportunity to have an analytic chat with Leonard. Perhaps you can find some reasonable explanation for the blood in his urine. If you prefer, I can have that chat with him.

Mr. James: Let me give it a try.

Edna: What is an "analytic chat"?

Dr. Louise: Let's wait for Dad to get back to us, Edna.

16:55
Mr. James: Dr. Louise, Leonard and I have had that chat. There is a reasonable explanation for the blood in his urine. I don't think we need to have further investigations.

Dr. Louise: Dad, I agree. His urine is clear now. We would reconsider the proposed tests if it happens again.

Mr. James: I appreciate the opportunity you provided to have Leonard talk to me. His only concern now is explaining all of this to his sister.

Dr. Louise: I expect that Leonard is going to get a few well-deserved verbal and head swats from her. Be sure to thank her for taking charge of her brother's situation.

Handover May 30, 16:00
Dr. John: Before Peter starts handover, can you update us on why the father didn't sign consent for the kidney x-ray? Edna told me that it was cancelled.

Dr. Louise: Oh, Dad came in as both of you were leaving. He is a chemistry professor. I suggested that he might want to have an analytic talk with Leonard. With a few well-constructed questions, he got Leonard to admit to what he had been doing just before the blood came out with his urine.

Dr. Peter: What made you go there?

Dr. Louise: Essentially the blood in the urine was a self-resolving event. The background is a fifteen-year-old, home alone, in bed, playing up a minor disability to stay home from school. The father got him to admit to what he was doing before the blood came out of his penis.

Edna: Yes, Louise, and on listening to this tale, this nurse is going to have a chat with her son.

Dr. Louise: What are you going to say to him?

Edna: I will ask him whether he wants to be traded in for a girl when he turns fifteen.

Dr. Louise: Don't wait to have that chat, Edna; but be careful what you wish for.

ENDNOTES

Chief Complaint – Blood in urine (fifteen-year-old male)

Vital Signs – Normal

Distractions: unusual complaint, little to find on examination

Snapshots of the vital history:

• A new analysis of the same history can lead to a different presumed diagnosis.

• Both invasive history and invasive procedure require consent.

- Is it too easy to ask for more investigations?
- When should we ask for the patient's assistance in determining the cause?
- When should we undertake a total review the vital history with the patient?

Two caregivers did not think to ask or they were reluctant to ask. What was the patient doing before blood appeared in his urine? The next caregiver weighed the risk of asking with the risk of an invasive dye injection and a high radiation dose. The arrival of the second next of kin and the third caregiver opens the opportunity to a new analysis of the history. Historical truth takes away the consequence of significant risks in the initial proposed investigations.

23

Bad Colour: Healthy Baby

Chief Complaint: Jaundice$^{\oplus}$
Emergency department team:
- Dr. Peter
- Dr. John
- Dr. Louise

Patient: Jane (fourteen-month-old)
Communication with:
- James (father)

Handover June 21, 16:00
Dr. Peter: Louise, that completes my handover. Triage has five patients. There are no expected transfers or ambulance arrivals. I will do a final review of each chart for each patient we have in each section. Could you take over the care of the patient John has just seen?

Dr. John: I have a baby in C4. Jane is a fourteen-month-old brought in by her father, James. The father's aunt, who is a retired nurse, is concerned that the baby is jaundiced. The aunt was quite insistent. Mother is away for three days and Dad is a bit overwhelmed with the feedings and the diaper changes.
Dr. Louise: What are the symptoms?

$^{\oplus}$**Jaundice** – yellow to yellow-green skin discoloration

Dr. John: None. It is just that father was worried that he was being told that the baby looked to have an awful colour.

Dr. Louise: What do you find on examination?

Dr. John: A picture of a chubby and playful fourteen-month-old who is jaundiced. Examination the chest and abdomen is normal.

Dr. Louise: What about her eyes?

Dr. John: They look normal to me. I am making out a blood test requisition. Besides a complete blood count and bilirubin$^{\oplus}$, do you want me to order any other liver function tests?

Dr. Louise: Have you checked the urine for bilirubin$^{\oplus}$?

Dr. John: We have placed a bag to collect a urine sample. Dad says that the stool colour is all over the place from bright green to orange to light brown.

Dr. Louise: John, I will come in to see the baby with you. What is your differential diagnosis?

Dr. John: Anything that blocks the biliary tract?

Dr. Louise: That would be very rare at this age especially in an otherwise well baby. You should add "or overwhelms the liver's ability to detoxify". Any medications?

$^{\oplus}$ **Bilirubin** – blood test to assess liver function

Dr. John: No.

Dr. Louise: Any breastfeeding?

Dr. John: At fourteen months?

Dr. Louise: I would not be surprised. Let's go and look at baby Jane. John, what are reasonable mileposts for feeding a growing baby?

Dr. John: Breast or formula with introduction of cereal at eight months, meat at ten months and vegetables at twelve months with fruit sometime thereafter.

16:25 Bedside Jane
Dr. Louise: Hi, Dad, I am told you have a healthy looking baby. I am Dr. Louise, the attending emergency physician. Dr. John, our resident has examined Jane and doesn't find any concerns. Let's just have another look. John, you have seen patients with jaundice before; what shade of yellow does baby Jane demonstrate?

Dr. John: More an orange than yellow or green.

Dr. Louise: And where is it most noticeable?

Dr. John: All over!

Dr. Louise: Yes, all over, but most noticeable on palms and soles and not as apparent in the white sclera[⊕] of the eyes.

James: What is the problem doctor?

[⊕] **Sclera** – the opaque white lining sheath of the eyeball

Dr. Louise: You and mother and baby Jane do not have anything to worry about. Young Jane is just demonstrating her fair skin and the effects of the introduction of squash and carrots into her diet within the last few months.

James: Should we stop those foods?

Dr. Louise: Absolutely not! Carry on and thank your aunt for being so observant.

James: She insisted that I listen to her.

Dr. John: Dr. Louise, what is the diagnosis?

Dr. Louise: John, the diagnosis is easy to remember: 'carotenemia'[⊕]. Look up your undergraduate pediatric lecture notes or just Google the word.

Dr. John: Now I will have to add diet history to my listening. Mr. James, can I take a picture of Jane? I will try to stump my resident colleagues with Jane's presentation.

ENDNOTES
Chief Complaint – Jaundice (fourteen-month-old baby)
Vital Signs – normal
Distractions: insistence of a respected family member, unusual appearance
Snapshots of the vital history:

[⊕] **Carotenemia** – a harmless transient clinical condition characterized by yellow pigmentation of the skin and increased beta-carotene levels in the blood

- Most prominent and least prominent locations help define the question of bad colour.
- Diet history is always relevant, especially in children.
- Caregivers, keep your class notes and Google close at hand.

A senior family member spells alarm to a baby's father about the baby's unusual colour. All physical signs point to a healthy baby. The father and the first caregiver do not have a rebuttal to the concern that has been put forward. A closer inspection and a standard diet history resolve the concern.

24

Overtaxed Heart: Use the Paddles

Chief Complaint: Fast irregular heart beat
Emergency department team:
- Dr. John
- Dr. Peter
- Dr. Louise
- Edward
- Dr. Richard (neurologist)
Communication with:
- Mr. Quinton (patient)
- Teresa (patient's niece)
- Sandra (patient's sister)
- CAT scan suite

Handover May 29, 16:00

Dr. John: Peter, before you start handover with Louise can you come back to see our Mr. Quinton in A3?

Dr. Peter: Is he OK to go home, John?

Dr. John: His pulse and blood pressure are fine. His sister has just arrived from the cemetery. She is concerned that Mr. Quinton seems a little confused, and is not speaking clearly.

Dr. Louise: Sister from the cemetery? What is the story, Peter?

16:05 Bedside Mr. Quinton

Dr. Peter: Mr. Quinton is a seventy-five-year-old male who came to us some two hours ago, having fainted at his wife's funeral. He presented in rapid atrial fibrillation⊕. He was adamant that we electrically convert him quickly so that he could at least attend the reception, if not the graveside prayers. He's had three bouts of atrial fibrillation over the past five years. One episode was remedied with intravenous medications over six hours. The other two episodes were taken care of with electric cardioversion. John and I provided 'conscious sedation⊕ and 100 joules⊕'. He successfully converted. Every ten minutes he has been asking to be discharged. We have been waiting for the sedation to wear off before testing how steady he is on his feet.

Edward: John and Peter, Mr. Quinton has slurred speech and marked weakness in his right arm and leg.

Dr. Peter: John, check those findings and complete a full neurological examination. Edward, please do a glucometer check and then prepare for a trip to the CAT scan suite. I will call them and send the requisition.

Dr. Louise: Do you want me to call the stroke team?

⊕**Atrial Fibrillation** – rhythm of continuous irregular beats in the upper heart chambers
⊕**Conscious Sedation** – combination of intravenous medications delivered in defined aliquot doses over specified time intervals to increase sedation and reduce pain for a patient while maintaining protective airway reflexes
⊕**Joules** – measurement of electric energy discharged by a defibrillator

Dr. Peter: Yes, please. Dr. Richards was just here a few minutes ago.

Edward: Will someone talk to Sandra, the sister, and Teresa, the niece?

Dr. Louise: Peter is coming into the room.

16:25 Main Desk
Dr. John: Dr. Richards, the neurologist, is looking at the CAT scan. He will be coming to explain to Mr. Quinton the pros and cons of trying to dissolve the clot in his brain.

16:35 Bedside Mr. Quinton
Dr. Richards: Mr. Quinton, Dr. Peter has asked us to assess you. You have had a stroke. The CAT scan confirms that there is a vessel blocked by a blood clot on the left side of your brain. We can try to dissolve that clot, and there is a good chance that we can improve the flow of blood. The risk is that we may cause you to bleed into your brain or from another vessel in your body. Are you on any blood thinners?

Mr. Quinton: No.

Dr. Richards: As Edward prepares the intravenous infusion, I will fill you in on the latest statistics for success, failure and complications of the treatment that we are proposing. We need to know if you have had any bleeding from your bowel or bladder, or any recent operations. We will need your consent.

Handover May 30, 08:00
Edward: John, how did Mr. Quinton do yesterday afternoon?

Dr. John: Most dramatic recovery. He is walking with some assistance this morning. His speech has completely resolved.

Edward: What a rotten triple-header for Mr. Quinton: wife's funeral, heart arrhythmia$^{\oplus}$ and a stroke all within a few hours.

Dr. Peter: Actually, those last two events were likely the result of the same play.

Edward: Why do you say that?

Dr. John: The history provided by Sandra, Mr. Quinton's sister, revealed that her brother was probably experiencing bouts of atrial fibrillation for at least the past week. She had tried to bring him to hospital when she found him holding on to furniture and the stair bannister with both hands on two separate occasions.

Dr. Peter: He probably formed a clot in his left atrial appendage$^{\oplus}$ over the past weeks. The cardioversion gave him a regular pulse and regular contractions, and the clot sprung out into his circulation.

Dr. John: He is scheduled for a cardiac echo$^{\oplus}$ this morning and carotid Dopplers$^{\oplus}$ this afternoon. The

---

$^{\oplus}$ **Arrhythmia** – abnormal heart beats in terms of rate and/or regularity

$^{\oplus}$ **Atrial Appendage** – an anatomic extension of the left and right atrial chambers of the heart

$^{\oplus}$ **Cardiac Echo and Carotid Dopplers** – non invasive ultrasound examination of heart cavities and neck vessels

$^{\oplus}$ **Anticoagulant** – medication to inhibit the formation of clots in the heart and blood vessels

neurology service is arranging his anticoagulant$^{\oplus}$ regimen.

Dr. Peter: We should have specifically asked Mr. Quinton about symptoms over the previous two weeks. Teresa, the niece, was unaware of any unusual symptoms, and Mr. Quinton only expressed today's symptoms and those of the distant past. If the sister had come with the patient, her version of the vital history might have triggered us to be cautious in using the electrical cardioversion mode of therapy. We understood why he wanted the fast therapeutic protocol. We didn't fully translate the background history.

ENDNOTES
Chief Complaint – Collapsed at wife's funeral (seventy-five-year-old male)

Vital Signs – irregular fast pulse

Distractions: social obligations for burial and reception, past treatment modalities

Snapshots of the vital history:

• A heart wanting to be somewhere else hides a threatening menace.

• Early discharge is a goal for both patient and caregivers.

• Closest 'next of kin' may have extra relevant information.

• Each treatment modality has specific recognized risks.

• Sound practised protocols seek to avoid known risks.

The caregivers do not pursue the detailed history with respect to duration of history. The available 'next of kin' is not aware of the past relevant history. The caregivers accept the patient's request for rapid resolution of symptoms. A serious complication occurs. The late arrival of another 'next of kin' confirms the details of the overlooked history.

25

The Trap: Never Thought To Ask

Chief Complaint: Persisting abdominal pain and diarrhea
Emergency department team:
- Dr. Peter
- Dr. Louise
- Dr. John
- Edward
- Microbiology consultant
- Pediatric resident

Communication with:
- Jason (patient)
- James (stepfather)
- Robert (father)

Handover June 23, 16:00

Dr. Peter: Louise, I completed handover with your co-attending for sections C and D. Welcome to section A. We have three admissions for Medicine and one for Neurosurgery. We are not expecting access to in-patient beds until tomorrow. There is a fifth patient for Neurosurgery, just intubated in A6, waiting for admission orders. There is one more patient in section A waiting for a report on her second acetaminophen level. Psychiatry is coming down to see her. John has been busy with the patients in section B; he needs to update me on one of them. Triage has four more patients to go to section B. John has one patient that we have not reviewed yet. There are no expected transfers or ambulance arrivals.

Dr. John: In B6, we have Jason, a fourteen-year-old boy with his stepfather, James. Jason has had abdominal cramps and diarrhea for eight days. He saw his family doctor three days ago. Stool specimens were collected. He stopped eating a week ago and has stopped drinking two days ago. Anything he takes by mouth makes the cramps and diarrhea worse.

Dr. Peter: Edward what are his present resting vital signs?

Edward: Pulse of 106, blood pressure 86 over 70; temperature normal. He is pale, has lost his skin turgor and is starting to look like a starved refugee.

Dr. Peter: John, anything on his history?

Dr. John: No fever. No chills. The symptoms were initially attributed to unrefrigerated food when he spent a weekend at his natural father's cottage three weekends ago. No one else is sick. The cottage doesn't have a fridge. They bring in bottled water. There is a family history of inflammatory bowel disease in an uncle.

Dr. Louise: Any blood work?

Dr. John: His haemoglobin is 110. His white cell count is normal. He has normal glucose and kidney function. The rest of his blood work is still pending. We are giving him two litres of normal saline and are planning to add some B vitamins and glucose to his IV.

Dr. Louise: Any travel, any medications, any contact with humans experiencing diarrhea? Any contact with animals that are sick? Has he had any food from restaurants or with large gathering of people? Any visits to retirement homes or hospitals?

Dr. John: No to all of those questions. There is a healthy dog and cat at home.

Dr. Louise: Any contact with turtles?

Dr. John: No.

Dr. Louise: What about the stool tests?

Dr. John: Yesterday's report was negative when the mother called the doctor's office this morning.

Dr. Louise: John, at eight days of symptoms and with this degree of dehydration, we should be admitting Jason. Let's call the pediatric service. Before you leave, can you check if there has been any significant travel in the last six months? Also check on his activities when he was at the cottage. I will call Microbiology and see if they will take a look at a fresh stool sample.

Handover June 24, 16:00
Dr. John: Louise, did you find anything about Jason's diarrhea?

Dr. Louise: Yes, the microbiologist had just reported on the initial stool specimen taken a few days ago ....

'Giardia cysts and trophozoites'[⊕].

[⊕] **Giardia cysts** – a resistant form of the parasite that can survive outside a human or animal body; causes spread of this disease (the parasites start growing and multiplying in the small intestine after the cysts are ingested)
[⊕] **Giardia trophozites** – the active mobile feeding stage of the Giardia lamblia parasite

Dr. John: Where did he catch that?

Edna: This morning the pediatric resident identified that Jason sometimes helps his natural father, Robert, set traps for the beavers that like to dam up the stream that runs into their lake.

Dr. John: We certainly did not hear that part of the history.

Dr. Louise: I agree, John. In this day and age, you really don't think of our patients setting up trap lines.

Dr. Peter: It's certainly not something that they readily admit to or consider it to be of consequence to their health. When contact with beavers is suspected as a cause of the intestinal symptoms, treatment can be initiated as soon as stool samples are taken.

Edward: Jason's admission process initially brought some opportunity for dialogue between the natural father and the stepfather. That quickly ended when the results of the stool sample were reported and the likely cause was determined to be water infested with beaver excrement. James, the stepfather, didn't want to listen any longer. He made a loud statement about animal cruelty as he was leaving the waiting room.

ENDNOTES
Chief Complaint – Persistent diarrhea (fourteen-year-old male)
Vital Signs – abnormal pulse, blood pressure and skin turgor

Distractions: Father and stepfather as 'next of kin'
Snapshots of the vital history:

- If you don't ask what you don't think is relevant you may not discover the diagnosis.
- Blended families introduce extra roadblocks to getting all of the vital history.
- Always pursue the results of previously ordered investigations.
- The search for sources of gastrointestinal infections needs to be exhaustive.
- Empirical therapy decisions can be made after sample gathering if suspicion is high.
- Cottages exist in different ecosystems than towns or cities.

Sometimes the history seems benign and further questions are fruitless. The patient, the 'next of kin' and the caregiver may not know or understand the relevance of the available history. Physical examination provides no specific diagnostic suggestions. Examination of the stool confirms what should have been gleaned from an appropriate investigative history.

26

Ninja Magic: Let's Listen To Our Heroes

Chief Complaint: Forehead laceration
Emergency department team:
- Dr. Louise
- Dr. Peter
- Edna
- Dr. John
- The Ninja heroes

Communication with:
- Jack (patient)
- James (father and patient)

Handover June 25, 09:00
Dr. Peter: We had a reasonable night shift, Louise. There are no known transfers expected. In Section A there are six of the seven admitted patients I faced at midnight. The seventh died, as expected, with prior DNR orders respected. We are told that there are no in-patient beds. I expect to be able to discharge two patients with food poisoning from the same meal in the same restaurant. C5 is waiting for the pharmacy to open so the patient can fill her pain prescription on the way home. She has a designated driver.

09:20

Edna: Peter, since you are finished giving handover, there is a double-header stitching in B3. Dad is asking for your attention. James and his three-year-old son, Jack, were racing their shopping cart in a grocery store parking lot and they hit a stop sign. They both received injuries; young Jack received his at the grocery store parking lot and Dad at our triage desk. I will let Jack and Dad explain.

09:22 Bedside Jack

Dr. Peter: Hi, Jack, I am Dr. Peter. I know your father, but I haven't met you before. What happened to you and Dad?

Jack: Got sticker on my hand!

Dr. Peter: What happened to your head?

Jack: Wow-wow head.

Dr. Peter: I see the nice bandage, Jack. Edna, will Jack need stitches?

Edna: Oh, big time!

Dr. Peter: How old are you, Jack?

Jack: Three fingers!

James: Jack, you are three and a half.

Dr. Peter: What happened, Dad?

James: We were in the grocery store parking lot. Found a stranded grocery cart, and decided to re-enact the Indianapolis 500. It was a lot of fun, but the team miscalculated around the stop sign: I went to the right and

Jack went to the left. Standing up, he was just tall enough to be clipped on the left side of his forehead. Needless to say, we didn't get the Saturday morning groceries for Mom.

Dr. Peter: But how did you get the cut on the top of your head?

James: That happened at triage. After the triage nurse put some anaesthetic ointment and a clean bandage on Jack's forehead, I asked the nurse to not show me the N-E-E-D-L-E.

Dr. Peter: I think I know where you are going with this, James. You and I have been through this discussion before.

James: She said, "Do you mean this N-E-E-D-L-E?" keeping it out of Jack's view as she thrust it in front of my face. The next thing she knew, I was on the floor and she was asking for a towel for the back of my head.

Dr. Peter: Are you OK now, James?

James: Yes, yes. Let's just get Jack fixed up.

Dr. Peter: So, Jack, can we fix your 'wowwe'?

Jack: Hurt?

Dr. Peter: Jack, we can take away the hurt if you can help us mix some magic.

Jack: Don't have magic!
Dr. Peter: Then we will need to get some from your best heroes. Who are some of your play heroes?

James: Dr. Peter, the Teenage Mutant Ninja Turtles are Jack's favourite heroes.

Dr. Peter: I have heard of them. They are super strong.

Jack: Super smart!

Dr. Peter: They are super smart, Jack. Can you help me to remember? Are they pretend heroes or are they real heroes?

Jack: Real!

Dr. Peter: Well let's use the Ninja magic then. First we will get Dad to turn around and lie upside down on the stretcher. You and I will call your hero friends to help us. Is Dad a good storyteller?

Jack: Naw, he forgets!

Dr. Peter: Dad can listen, and then you and Dad can tell Mom the Ninja magic story when you go home. Dr. John is our helper here. He just came in because he heard that the Ninjas were in here. He says that he can't see them? Jack, where are our Ninjas?

Jack: In our brain!

Dr. Peter: Yes, Jack. Let's plan for the first Ninja. Think of who you want to be the first Ninja to help us. Edna is going to put a towel under your head and we can put your stinky toes on top of Dad's tummy.
Jack: Not stinky!

Dr. Peter: Not as bad as Daddy's. I think we will put some more towels over Dad's feet. Jack, you can hold Dad's hands upside down. Now Jack, whenever we do something for your wowee, we will tell you. What you have to do is answer the questions so that the Ninja that you choose can use his powers to help us fix your head. Jack, can you tell Dr. John the names of the Ninjas?

Jack: Raphael...Michelangelo...Leonardo... and, I forget.

Dr. Peter: John, can you help us out?

Dr. John: No, I forget too.

James: Donatello?

Jack: Yes. Donatello.

Dr. Peter: Jack, tell us, who is the silliest Ninja?

Jack: Don't know.

Dr. Peter: What does Dad have to say?

James: Leonardo?

Dr. Peter: Yep. Jack, do you know what Leonardo is famous for?

Jack: No?

Dr. Peter: Leonardo was the first person to build a catapult and design a helicopter.
Jack: What is 'catput'?

Dr. Peter: A catapult throws big stones to break down the walls of the castles. I am using a tiny catapult to send some medicine in to clear up all this yucky blood. Can you hear the splashing when the medicine hits the strong castle wall on your head? Five catapults should break this castle wall. Finished three catapults. Now four catapults. Finished this part.

Jack: Leonardo finished magic?

Dr. Peter: Yes, Jack. I think we can use the next Ninja now. Who would you like?

Jack: Raphael?

Dr. Peter: Good choice, Jack. Raphael was a famous painter. His mother was always angry with him. Do you know why?

Jack: Raphael paint!

Dr. Peter: Messy, messy; he would never wash his hands. Do you wash your hands when Mommy asks? Edna is going to give us some special water to use in a squirt gun. Maybe we can let you take it home to show mom. Dad, can Jack keep our squirt gun?

Jack: Yes, Dad? Toy squirt gun, Dad!

Dr. Peter: Hey, Jack, this squirt gun washed out some red paint. Where do you think that came from?

Jack: Stop sign red!

Dr. Peter: Now Jack, who will be the third Ninja to help us?

Jack: Donatello!

Dr. Peter: Good choice, Donatello was a real magician. He could pull anything he wanted out of a basket by snapping his fingers. We are going to use some of that magic by going into the basket that I see and pulling blue thread out. You will hear the snap each time I tie one of the threads. I am just learning to use Donatello's magic, so I will have to do the snapping eight times. What? You want to take the snap scissors home too? Don't think so, Jack. Donatello and I will need them in the next room. Bugs Bunny was cutting carrots with a sharp knife and he cut his thumb. Do we call it a thumb on a bunny or do we call it a paw?

Jack: Thumb!

Dr. Peter: Jack, we have had the help from three of the brave Ninjas and we are almost finished. Tell me about the last one?

Jack: Michelangelo!

Dr. Peter: Michelangelo is really special for two reasons. He can make giant pieces of stone look like anything he wants. Dad, what is the second reason Michelangelo is a super special Ninja?

James: I think he is the boss of the Ninjas.

Dr. Peter: Jack, I think your head is just the shape that Michelangelo would want. Who is the boss at home? Dad?
Jack: Mommy!

Dr. Peter: Edna just said that Mommy is here to see you. Before Mom comes in, you need to know that your Ninja friends have asked you a special question.

Jack: What question?

Dr. Peter: The Ninja leader wants you to join their team. We need to give Michelangelo two answers. Number one: are you brave?

Dr. John: Jack is the bravest!

Dr. Peter: Number two: are you strong? Edna and Dr. John are nodding yes. You have passed the Ninja team test, Jack. Michelangelo wants you to wear part of their uniform. Do you know what the Ninja's wear on their head? Jack, do you know what it is called?

Jack: Don't member.

Dr. Peter: A bandana! Edna do you think Jack deserves a Ninja bandana on his head.

Edna: You bet!

Dr. Peter: Jack, what does Michelangelo say to his team when they are going out on a mission?

Jack: Be careful!

Dr. Peter: John, I will look at Dad while you take Jack out to Mom. No Ninja magic for Dad. Just one stitch to his scalp. Edna, can Dad have a bandana too?

Edna: No magic, no bandana!

James: Please, no needles in sight.

09:40 Main Desk

Dr. Peter: Edna, why do you have that puzzled look on your face?

Edna: How can such a brave three-year-old come from such a wimpy father?

Dr. Peter: Actually, Edna, there are only a very few people in this department and in this community who really know Jack's father. Can I explain?

Edna: I'm sure you will.

Dr. Peter: James is the chief trainer of the provincial police SWAT team[⊕]. He has earned the reputation of being a real life Ninja. He is undoubtedly the toughest officer known to the provincial police force.

Edna: And he is scared of needles?

Dr. Peter: The paradox still remains for James. Threaten him with guns and knives and he can stand his ground; show him a tiny needle and you will need to pick him up off the floor. As a child he had allergies and received allergy shots almost daily until he was nine. It would take two adults to contain him each time he was to get a needle.

Edna: A real, earned phobia.

Dr. Peter: He grew out of his allergies, but not his unrealistic fear of needles. We have had the discussion of

---

[⊕] **SWAT team** – special weapons and tactics team

getting therapy in the past. I brought it up again today. He has agreed to get some counselling and deconditioning therapy. He has his eye on a post in the narcotics division.

Edna: He needs to find out how he can listen to and use the Ninja magic in his head.

ENDNOTES
Chief Complaint – Forehead laceration (three-year-old boy)
Vital Signs -normal
Distractions: age, injury, father's phobia
Snapshots of the vital history:

- Adults tell stories; Children live stories.
- Active story telling can distract us from fear of the unknown.
- Our selected heroes are ready to share their talents with us.
- A child can actively assist in directing the story telling.
- What can we learn from a three-year-old in active dialogue with his heroes?
- We need to ask our heroes/colleagues to share their talents with us.
- Guided Imagery is more than magic.
- Guided imagery or conscious sedation – what and who makes the choice?
- A father may need to work at learning what comes natural to his child.

A child joins in the telling of a story about the abilities of his fearless and smart play heroes. The father and caregivers are invited to participate. There is a role for each hero. The role accepted by the child expedites the work of the caregivers. An invitation to join the band of play heroes is the reward of recognition of this child's innate talents.

27

Who Is Listening: Mudpiles and Beyond

Chief Complaint: Intoxication
Emergency department team:
- Dr. Peter
- Dr. John
- Dr. Louise
- Edna

Patients: Twin thirteen-year-old boys
Communication with:
- James (father)
- Carol (mother)

Handover June 27, 08:00

Dr. Peter: Louise, our major concern this morning is with the two patients in A7 and A8. We have thirteen-year-old twin boys who thought that they would celebrate the end of classes with a little tequila last night. They were brought in early this morning by their parents, James and Carol. When Mom and Dad came home at 11 p.m. they realized that the boys were drunk. The boys admitted to creating some fancy drinks. Two inches of a twenty-five-ounce bottle of tequila were missing. The parents put them to bed, but had to get up twice in the night because of their vomiting. By 6 a.m. this morning, the parents began to get worried because the boys were completely out of it: they were   confused,   had   slurred   speech,   and   were uncoordinated. The parents became frightened and brought both of them in to Emergency. They were concerned that there may also have been some drugs involved.

Dr. John: On arrival, it was evident that we had really sick cookies with rapid respiratory rates and rapid pulses. They had minimal mumbled verbal responses to painful stimuli.

Dr. Louise: What did the blood work show?

Dr. John: It revealed the expected classical presentation of high anion gap$^{\oplus}$ acidosis plus a high osmolar gap$^{\oplus}$.

Dr. Peter: There was some significant confusion as to how this occurred. The initial blood ethanol levels were not seriously elevated. In cross checking the MUDPILES acronym, the only lead was the alcohol ingestion. On further questioning of the parents, James mentioned buying some absolute alcohol across the border a few months ago, but quickly claimed that he had distributed his entire last haul to his buddies. John wisely asked the father to go home and check the garage and house for any containers of alcohol or antifreeze. James found that one of two containers of antifreeze had been opened and not properly recapped, but it seemed full.

$^{\oplus}$ **Anion Gap** – the difference between the measured cations (positively charged ions – e.g. sodium and potassium) and the anions (negatively charged ions – e.g. chloride and bicarbonate) in the serum of the blood sample
$^{\oplus}$ **Osmolar gap** –the difference between measured and calculated osmolality in the serum of a blood sample

Dr. John: Treatment has been started: intravenous fluids, bicarbonate, intravenous alcohol and fomepizole⊕. The boys are now en route to the Intensive Care Unit.

Dr. Louise: If you want, I can start seeing the patients that the triage desk is bringing to Section B. Let me know when you want to complete handover.

Dr. Peter: John and I need to make our rounds and then we will come back and fill you in on further details of the patients we will handover to your care.

Handover June 29, 08:00
Dr. Louise: Peter, before today's handover, how did the boys with the suspected antifreeze poisoning fare?

Dr. Peter: They were both out of Intensive Care Unit this morning and probably will be going home tomorrow. It will be the longest drunk these boys will ever experience. Also the cheapest!

Edna: The most expensive for the taxpayer.

Dr. Louise: Any idea as to what made them drink antifreeze?

Dr. John: It's unbelievable. One of the twins had heard the father talking to his buddy about how he had taken six five-litre containers full of antifreeze across the border, and how cleverly he had drained four of the containers and refilled them with ninety proof ethanol and just the right amount of food colouring. He boasted that he saved about three hundred dollars with his ingenious

---

⊕ **Fomepizole** – an antidote in confirmed or suspected methanol or ethylene glycol poisoning; used alone or in combination with ethanol

switch. The twins did not realize that the father had also left two intact five-litre antifreeze containers in the garage. They thought it was the contraband alcohol. They took out a sample and replaced the withdrawn amount with coloured water.

Dr. Louise: Like father, like sons!

Dr. Peter: Selective listening on their part.

Dr. Louise: What made you focus on the antifreeze, ethylene glycol?

Dr. John: The M.U.D.P.I.L.E.S. acronym can help you navigate uncharted waters; the acronym has stood the test of time. We went over the list of possibilities and the only one that made sense was the antifreeze.

Dr. Peter: John, can you update us on any recent revisions in the 'mudpiles' acronym?

Dr. John: I read up on it last night. M.U.D.P.A.I.L.E.S.// M.U.D.P.I.L.E.R.S.// C.U.T.E. D.I.M.P.L.E.S are all easy to remember, so there's no need to waste time trying to hunt down clues to the cause of the metabolic acidosis. I have made a cue card to keep close at hand.

Dr. Peter: Share it with us, John!

Dr. John: I have made some copies.

High Anion Gap Acidosis:
<u>*M*</u> **ethanol (wood alcohol and windshield wiper antifreeze)**
<u>*U*</u> **remia (kidney failure)**

D iabetic ketoacidosis

P ropylene glycol (solvent for parental medications)

I soniazid, Iron

L actic Acidosis (infection and dead tissue from no blood flow)

E thylene glycol (antifreeze), Ethanol

S alicylates (aspirin products), Short Bowel Syndrome,

Latest revisions and additions:

PAILES A…alcoholic ketoacidosis

PAILERS R…rhabdomyolysis

CUTE DIMPLES C…cyanide T…toluene P…phenformin

ENDNOTES

Chief Complaint – 'Intoxication' (twin thirteen-year-old boys)

Vital Signs – severely abnormal

Distractions: abnormal vital signs, no known cause, two patients

Snapshots of the vital history:

• Accepted acronyms can point the caregiver in the right direction.

• Alcohol has many faces.

• Deadly poisons are never far away from idle hands.

• When adults brag, do they care to know who is listening?

Sometimes history is momentarily suspended to initiate lifesaving resuscitation and calculations of needed life sustaining therapy. There is always a history that needs to be traced down. The delayed history will help

221

confirm that the aggressive therapy is appropriate and worth the risk undertaken.

28

Tuned In: No Guarantee

Chief Complaint: Hearing voices
Emergency department team:
- Dr. Peter
- Dr. John
- Dr. Louise
- Edward

Patient: Rodney
Communication with:
- Mr. James (father)
- Doreen (sister)

Handover October 07, 08:00

Dr. Peter: Louise, let's complete the handover for this morning. Triage has eight patients. There is an eighteen-year-old motor vehicle accident victim with chest pain and a fractured leg coming in for the Trauma Team. He is expected to arrive in twenty minutes. John and I have one patient to handover.

Dr. John: In D4, we have Rodney, a twenty-year-old male with his family, waiting for a psychiatry assessment. Rodney is a second-year university student in Toronto. He has unexpectedly come home from his classes. Last year he just managed to pass his year; he lost his academic scholarship. This year he has switched from biochemistry to botany.

Dr. Louise: Why is he here this morning?

Dr. John: Two days ago, without notice, Rodney returned home by bus; the only explanation given to his parents was that "he was needed". The parents noted that he was not eating and not talking much. After repeated questions, he is now telling his parents and us that "the university radio station had told him to go home to get direct instructions from the air force base command".

Dr. Louise: What has happened since he came home?

Dr. John: He has kept to his room for the past thirty-six hours. When Mom and Dad came home from a neighbour's visit late last evening, they noticed that Rodney was sitting on the roof in his pyjamas looking at the sky. Initially he did not respond to their questions, but then he asked them to be quiet so that he could better make out the instructions he needed to receive. They were up all night with him walking in circles in the family room; he insisted on keeping the patio doors wide open. They finally convinced him to join them in their trip to the hospital so they could get some help or instructions as to what they should do.

Dr. Louise: Any past history of similar episodes? Any history of drug use?

Dr. John: There is no apparent history of drug use. His only past medical history is wisdom teeth extractions two years ago. He is not on any medications and has no history of head trauma, fever or unusual behaviour in the past. Rodney seems oriented to person and place but not to time. He denies anxiety, worry or depression. He looks somewhat sullen; there is a sardonic smirk in his facial expressions, and he has a dismissive body language. He answers about one in five questions. His explanation is that he can't be bothered and he needs to concentrate on getting the right message. He says that his earphones are now dialled-in to pick up the instructions from the command post at the air force base.

Edward: His sister, Doreen, is in her senior year of high school. She is crying outside the room. She is overwhelmed by her big brother's actions. He is not relating to her. She does not exist as far as Rodney is concerned. She is asking us to check if he is taking any drugs. She is unaware of any personal romantic friendships. She declares that, "He is totally different; it's hard to accept that he has the same face but has a devil's smile."

Dr. John: Rodney is pacing the floor. The security guards want to leave. The psychiatry resident is coming to see him. Rodney is not aggressive, and has accepted soup and sandwiches. His eyes are constantly darting in all directions.

Edward: Rodney wants to go out for a smoke, but his sister says that he doesn't smoke. He wants the overhead paging system turned off because it is interfering with the messages coming in to him.

Dr. Louise: What do the messages say?

Dr. John: "Prepare to take charge" is the only response I get from Rodney. I have decided to complete an 'involuntary psychiatry consultation form' on him. Even though he has been cooperative, he is worrisome. The parents had a hard time coaxing him off the steep roof last night; all of a sudden, he finally decided just to jump down some seven feet. We get the feeling that he is holding back on telling us what the voice or voices are actually instructing him to do. There is enough concern that he may suddenly bolt, and we will be playing catch-up with a six-foot, determined and directed young man.

Handover October 11, 08:00

Dr. John: What was the follow-up on the university student getting instructions from air force command?

Dr. Louise: First Onset Psychosis! He is responding well to medication. There is discussion about him returning to classes next term.

Edward: Were there any prior warnings of the psychosis?

Dr. Louise: The sister told the psychiatry resident that when she drove him to university this September, Rodney had frightened her during the car trip. He suddenly stopped her conversation in mid-sentence, saying that he wanted to hear what was being announced on the car radio. The radio was not on. Initially she felt offended, but later chalked it up to the fact that maybe she was talking too much, and "it was my brother's weird way of getting me to be quiet". Doreen regrets that she so clearly misinterpreted the significance of her brother's spoken words.

Dr. John: Edward, tell Louise what Dad's comment was upon leaving the emergency department last evening.

Edward: I've never heard a parent say this before: "You know that you need to feed and take care of your children; you know that you have to protect them. However, no one reminds you that they don't come with a warranty."

ENDNOTES

Chief Complaint – 'Hearing voices' (twenty-year-old male)

Vital Signs – normal; baffling behaviour and weird answers to questions

Distractions: cooperative, security guards want to leave

Snapshots of the vital history:

- A captured mind induces agony for family members.
- How should we react when our conversation is unexplainably cut short?
- How should caregivers respond to a patient's demand to "go out for a smoke"?
- Parents are not provided a warranty.

A never-ending awake nightmare for the family is transpiring. Each question produces answers that frighten all members. Reality is broken. The present and the past are searched for explanations and evidence. Each family member forever carries an added burden. The first step has been taken along an uncharted path for a patient and his family.

29

Something Is Not Right: House Call

Chief Complaint: Low blood sugar
Emergency department team:
- Dr. Peter
- Edna
- Pharmacist: Mr. Randolph Scott
- Dr. John
- Medicine resident: Dr. Ken Jacob
- Paramedic
- Dr. Louise
- Ward Clerk

Communication with:
- David/Dave (patient)
- Mr. James Stone (father)

Handover November 28 16:00
Dr. Peter: Louise, go ahead and get started seeing patients. John and I have just completed a walk around the department. I will be ready as soon as I answer a phone message from a pharmacist who wants to double-check a prescription I wrote for insulin.

Edna: Line 231 is for you, Peter.
Dr. Peter: This is Dr. Peter from General Hospital Emergency Department. You have a question about a prescription?

Pharmacist: Yes, this is Randolph Scott at City Pharmacy. We have an insulin prescription written by you for a Dave Stone. We are not sure if it reads 25 or 35 units at bedtime. Patient said 35 and we filled the prescription. Today our pharmacy assistant wants to check with you before she enters the data on this new patient into our system.

Dr. Peter: Sorry, Randolph, I don't recall writing that prescription, and I don't recall that patient. When was the date, and are you sure it was my name?

Pharmacist: It has your name and your signature on your department's prescription pad template. The date was November 14.

Dr. Peter: Let me look up the name and the date in our medical record system. I will call you back.

16:15
Dr. Peter: Dr. Peter calling. Could I speak to Mr. Scott? Randolph, I am returning your call about that insulin prescription. The only patient with the last name of "Stone" that I saw was three days earlier, and the prescription was for a diuretic for a "James Stone" living at 123 Leader Road.

Pharmacist: This prescription is for a "David Stone" at apartment 36, 1414 Johnson Street.

Dr. Peter: Sorry, we don't have any record of such a patient.
Pharmacist: Could your house staff have filled out the prescription under your name?

Dr. Peter: No. They would sign it with their own names.

Pharmacist: How about a medical student? Could it be for a staff member or an acquaintance or a family member of one of your patients?

Dr. Peter: I would recall such a request for a patient who was not registered. I would need some basis to determine both the type of insulin and the dose. Randolph, can you just wait a moment? Our resident, Dr. John, is just pointing out on the computer screen that a David Stone was admitted to hospital two evenings ago. Let me check into this a little further. I will call you back after I do some more investigating. John, do you know anything about David Stone's admission?

Dr. John: Only what I heard from the senior emergency medicine resident at handover yesterday morning. David is a new outpatient clinic nurse. He came in for his second episode of fainting and confusion. They were concerned about his low blood sugar. I believe they are working him up for an endocrine disorder. Edna may know more.

Dr. Peter: Edna, do you know which Internal Medicine resident is covering the floor?

Edna: Dr. Ken Jacob on pager 3335.

Dr. Peter: Thanks Edna, I will call him now. Ken, it's Peter in the emergency department. Our emergency medicine resident, John, tells me that you have a David or Dave Stone admitted on your ward. Would it be possible for me to come talk to him?

Dr. Jacob: It would, but he is not here. He asked to go home to pick up some reading material and his computer. We are planning to keep him for a few more days, and he doesn't have any family in town. He needs to be back by 7:00 pm when his twenty-four-hour urine collection is due.

Dr. Peter: But there is a father listed on his emergency admission record. He lives in town.

Ken: Hadn't noticed that. Come up to see him after 7 pm if you want to talk to him.

Dr. Peter: Not if I see him sooner!

Dr. John: What did you mean by that, Peter?

Dr. Peter: Edna, were you here when David Stone came in two nights ago?

Edna: Yes, just going off shift. He responded well to the glucose push. I understand he needed another bolus a few hours later. I was not aware of the fact that he was a nurse. He was quite confused. I left soon after I gave the first bolus of glucose. What is your concern, Peter?

Dr. Peter: I am going to call his father's number. Can I use the charge nurse's office to make this call? I don't think I want our conversation overheard.

16:40 Charge Nurse Office
Dr. Peter: James Stone, this is Dr. Peter from the emergency department. I saw you about two weeks ago

and changed your diuretic medication. Has that helped your ankle swelling?

Mr. Stone: Yes, thanks.

Dr. Peter: Have you followed up with your own doctor?

Mr. Stone: Yes, last week.

Dr. Peter: Good. I have another question for you: do you have a son named David?

Mr. Stone: Why yes, Dave just started working at your hospital. Why do you ask?

Dr. Peter: There is some confusion about a prescription. Is your son a diabetic?

Mr. Stone: No, he is in excellent health. He takes good care of his diet and activity. He knows that I am a Type 2 diabetic. I talk to him every few days. He runs errands for me now that my vision is poor. Are you sure you have the right person? Maybe the prescription was for me and they mixed up the name.

Dr. Peter: Are you on insulin, Mr. Stone?

Mr. Stone: No, just oral tablets.

Dr. Peter: Have you talked to your son today?

Mr. Stone: No, he usually phones me before supper, but we haven't talked in a few days. I thought this call was going to be from him.

Dr. Peter: Mr. Stone, can you give him a call and ask him to contact me at the hospital? The operator will page me.

Mr. Stone: Actually, I have called him twice this afternoon, just before you called. Don't think he's home. Could he be doing an extra shift at work?

Dr. Peter: If you do get a hold of him, please ask him to call the hospital operator and page Dr. Peter. Thanks, Mr. Stone.

16:55 Main Desk

Dr. Peter: John, are you finished reviewing your patients for handover?

Dr. John: Yes. Can I do anything for you?

Dr. Peter: 1414 Johnson is only two blocks away. I won't be able to rest until I resolve this prescription issue. Can you take a few minutes? We can both check in on this David or Dave.

Dr. John: What if he is not home?

Dr. Peter: I am concerned enough that I would ask the building superintendent to check the apartment.

Dr. John: Why not just phone him?

Dr. Peter: His father has received no answer on two calls today.

17:25 Main Desk

Edna: Paramedic patch on line one.

Paramedic: Thirty-year-old male, unconscious; dextrose stick⊕ of 'one point five'. Received 50cc's of 50% glucose; minimal response. Pulse 42 and weak; systolic blood pressure 90. Two doctors accompanying.

Dr. Louise: What is the expected time of arrival?

Paramedic: ETA⊕ is three minutes.

Edna: Let's clear A2. I will get another syringe of 50 per cent glucose ready.

17:45 Resuscitation Room A2
Dr. Peter: Louise, John and I can now start today's delayed handover with this new (to us) but recycled inpatient who already has an in-patient bed but probably on the wrong service.

Dr. Louise: I was wondering whether you two just wanted to escape from the department.

Dr. Peter: It must be twenty years since I last did a house call.

17:50 Main Desk
Ward Clerk: "This is General Hospital Emergency Department calling. We are looking for any relative of a David Stone. Do you know how we can contact his family?"
ENDNOTES
Review of emergency department communications:
Chief Complaint – Low blood sugar (adult male)

⊕ **Dextrose Stick** – Reading of glucose measurement on a glucometer when a drop of blood is analysed
⊕ **ETA** – expected time of arrival

Snap Shots from the vital history:

- Routine check of a prescription raises a flag!
- What we are hearing does not make sense!
- Listening to more history suggests a disaster in the making!
- Do emergency caregivers make house calls?
- A criminal act or repeated desperate pleas for help?
- We need to put in a call to the 'next of kin'!

Red flags in the emergency department setting require a stop of action to consider the "what, why, when and who". History can be found from indirect sources outside of the patient and 'next of kin'. Red flags tell us that something is not right. Danger lurks around the next uncovered piece of information. The reason for the flags must be ascertained. This is vital history that cannot be put aside for another time, another visit.

Medical Literature References

1. The value of history and goals of care with code status; even in an emergency setting. Irfan A; Hublikar S; Cho JH; Hill J. BMJ Case Reports. 2013.

2. All info is good info. Seek & incorporate all available patient information. Heightman AJ. Journal of Emergency Medical Services. 39(4): 10, 2014 Apr. [Editorial]

3. Missed and delayed diagnoses in the emergency department: a study of closed malpractice claims from 4 liability insurers. Kachalia A; Gandhi TK; Puopolo AL; Yoon C; Thomas EJ; Griffey R; Brennan TA; Studdert DM. Annals of Emergency Medicine. 49(2): 196-205, 1997 Feb.

4. Do not forget to listen to the ambulance crew and the spouse. Calle P; De Schyver D. European Journal of Emergency Medicine: 1998, 5, 2, 269-271.

5. Rosen's Emergency Medicine – Concepts and Clinical Practice. 8th edition John A Marx, Robert J. Hockberger, Ron M. Walls; August 15, 2012.

6. Using the synergy model of patient care in understanding the lived emergency department experiences of patients, family members and their nurses during critical illness: a phenomenological study. Cypress B S; DCCN – Dimensions of Critical Care Nursing. 32(6): 310-21, 2013 Nov-Dec.

7. Improving parent-provider communication in the pediatric emergency department: results from the clear and concise communication campaign. Porter SC; Johnston P; Parry G; Damian F; Hoppa EC; Stack AM. Pediatric Emergency Care. 27(2): 75-80, 2011 Feb.

8. The Passion and the Peril: Storytelling in Medicine. Ofri D. Academic Medicine, 2015:1.

9. Doctor as story-listener and storyteller. Schwartz R. Can Fam Physician. 2007 Aug; 53(8): 1288–1289.

10. Medical Readers' Theater: A Guide and Scripts Edited by Todd L Savitt, University of Iowa Press Iowa City, Iowa 52242 ISBN 0-87745-799-9.

Selected Readings for Emergency Department Listeners

Every Patient Tells a Story: Medical Mysteries and the Art of Diagnosis – Lisa Saunders ☐ Harmony; Reprint edition (Sept. 21 2010). ISBN-**10:** 0767922476 ☐ ISBN-**13:** 978-0767922470

Patient Listening; A Doctor's Guide – Editor Loreen Herwaldt. University of Iowa Press, 1 edition (April 15, 2008)   ISBN-10:1587296527☐ISBN-13:   978-1587296529

Communication in Everyday Life: A Survey of Communication – Steve Duck, David T. McMahan. SAGE Publications, Second edition (January 15, 2014) ISBN-**10:** 145225978X ☐ ISBN-**13:** 978-1452259789

Reflective Practice – Gillie Bolton. SAGE Publications, 4 edition (Aug. 26 2014) ISBN-10: 144628235X ☐ ISBN-**13:** 978-1446282359

Doctors in the Making: Memoirs and Medical Education Suzanne Poirier March 16, 2009 University of Iowa Press, 1 edition (March 16, 2009) ISBN-10: 1587297922 ISBN-13: 978-1587297922

Between the Heartbeats: **Poetry and Prose by Nurses** (Cambridge Language Education) Cortney Davis (Editor), Judy Schaefer (Editor), Joanne Trautmann Banks (Foreword) ☐ University of Iowa Press; Rev

edition (November 1, 1995) ISBN-10: 0877455171
ISBN-13: 978-0877455172

The Orange Wire Problem and Other Tales From the Office – David H. Watts. University of Iowa Press; 1 edition (April 28, 2009) ISBN-10: 1587298007 ISBN-**13**: 978-1587298004

Grammar Lessons – Michele Morano. University of Iowa Press, 1 edition (January 1, 2014) ISBN-10: 1609382641 ☐ ISBN-13: 978-1609382643

The Checklist Manifesto; How to Get Things Right – Atul Gawande☐ Picador; Reprint edition (Jan. 4, 2011) ☐ ISBN-10: 0312430000 ☐ ISBN-**13**: 978-0312430009

After The Error: Speaking Out About Patient Safety to Save Lives – Susan B. McIver/ Robin Wyndham Published: April 1, 2013 ECW Press ISBN – 10: 1770411100. ISBN – 13: 9781770411104

Interference – Michelle Berry. ECW Press, 1 edition (Aug. 1 2014) ☐ ISBN: 1770411984

La Pieta of the Emergency Room – Brian Deady. Canadian Medical Association Journal; October 14, 2003; 169(8).

Bloodletting & Miraculous Cures – Vincent Lam. 2005 Anchor Canada; 1 edition (Sept. 26 2006) ☐ ISBN-10: 0385661444 ☐ ISBN-13: 978-0385661447

The Night Shift – Brian Goldman. HarperCollins Publishers Ltd (Sept 2, 2011)
☐ ISBN-10: 1554683920 ☐ ISBN-13: 978-1554683925

The Floater's Log – Ron Krome. Publishamerica Inc (Oct 1, 2007)☐ ISBN-10: 1424182824 ☐ ISBN-13: 978-1424182824

Collection of Short Stories – Margaret Lewis. Austin Macauley Publishers Ltd: 1 edition (Oct.31, 2014). ISBN -10: 1849634599. ISBN -13: 978-1849634595

Glossary of Medical Terms

This glossary of terms is provided to assist the non-health care reader in understanding more fully the interactive dialogue that is occurring in the emergency department among patients, 'next of kin' and caregivers in each encounter where a "Call to Listen" is needed. It is not intended to explain specific terms with respect to the significance of symptoms, therapeutic decisions, or the determination of a definitive diagnosis.

Acetaminophen – pain and fever medication (also under brand names of 'tylenol' and 'paracetamol')

Adenopathy – swollen lymph glands

Anaesthesia – the specialty that supports airway, breathing, pain and consciousness

Angiogram – injection of dye into an artery to make the shape, contour and contents of the artery visible

Anion Gap – the difference between the measured cations (positively charged ions – e.g. sodium and potassium) and the anions (negatively charged ions – e.g. chloride and bicarbonate) in the serum of the blood sample

Anticoagulant – medication to inhibit the formation of clots in the heart and blood vessels

Aplastic Anemia – reduced number of blood cells (red, white and platelet) due to disease of bone marrow

Arrhythmia – abnormal heart beats in terms of rate and/or regularity

Arterial Blood Gas – sample of blood from an artery for the measurement of acid base balance (pH and the concentration of oxygen, carbon dioxide and bicarbonate]

Atrial Appendage – an anatomic extension of the left and right atrial chambers of the heart

Atrial Fibrillation – rhythm of continuous irregular beats in the upper heart chambers

Bilirubin – blood test to assess liver function

Bundle Branch Block – appearance on the electrocardiogram that identifies the location of a defect in the conduction system of the heart

Carbon Dioxide Detector – measures the amount of carbon dioxide in the exhaled breath

Cardiac Echo and Carotid Dopplers – non- invasive ultrasound examination of heart cavities and neck vessels

Cardiology – Specialty for heart disorders

Carotenemia – a harmless transient clinical condition characterized by yellow pigmentation of the skin and increased beta-carotene levels in the blood

Cath Lab – (Cardiac Catheter Laboratory) A special hospital unit where invasive assessment of heart function and necessary procedures are performed using catheters that gain access through extremity arteries and veins

CAT scan – computer assisted tomography scan [also **CT scan**]

Chloramphenicol – useful broad-spectrum antibiotic available since 1949 for the treatment of a number of bacterial infections

Conscious Sedation – combination of intravenous medications delivered in defined aliquot doses over specified time intervals to increase sedation and reduce pain for a patient while maintaining protective airway reflexes

Coroner – a government official (usually a qualified physician) who investigates, confirms and certifies the occurrence and the cause of death of an individual within a jurisdiction

CPR – cardio-pulmonary resuscitation

Creatinine – a blood test, which is used to evaluate kidney function; a by-product of creatine, which is involved with muscle energy metabolism; filtered from the blood by the kidneys and excreted into urine

Cystoscopy – visual examination of the inside of the urinary bladder with a special instrument
Dextrose Stick – reading of glucose measurement on a glucometer when a drop of blood is analysed

Diuretic – medication that increases fluid loss through its action on the kidneys

DNA – deoxyribonucleic acid; responsible for storing and transferring genetic information

DNR – Do Not Resuscitate

DOA – Dead On Arrival

ECG – electrocardiogram

Ejection Fraction – the proportion of blood in the left ventricle pushed out with each contraction

EMS – emergency medical services

ETA – expected time of arrival

Exsanguinate – death from massive or continuous blood loss

Femur – upper leg bone

Fomepizole – an antidote in confirmed or suspected methanol or ethylene glycol poisoning; used alone or in combination with ethanol

Fractured spleen – the breaking of the spleen causing escape of blood into the abdomen

Giardia cysts – a resistant form of the parasite that can survive outside a human or animal body; causes spread of this disease (the parasites start growing and multiplying in the small intestine after the cysts are ingested) **Giardia trophozites** – the active mobile feeding stage of the Giardia lamblia parasite

Globulin (Rabies Immune Globulin) – used together with rabies vaccine to prevent infection caused by the rabies virus; works by providing the needed antibodies until the patient can produce sufficient antibodies against the rabies virus.

Glucometer – measuring instrument for 'stat' (immediate) blood glucose (sugar) level

Greenstick fracture – a break in a long bone (usually a child's) where the bark of the bone is buckled but there is no gap at the fracture site

HCG – human chorionic gonadotropin hormone produced by the placental cells following implantation of fertilized egg

Hematologist – specialist in blood disorders

Heparin – injectable anticoagulant (blood thinner) used to treat and prevent blood clots in the veins, arteries, or lung

HIV – Human Immunodeficiency Virus; causes AIDS (Acquired Immune Deficiency Syndrome)

Hyperthyroidism – Overactive thyroid gland producing a constellation of symptoms and some physical signs including susceptibility to bone fractures

Idiosyncratic – pertaining to or rationalizing that there is something peculiar and not understood about the interaction with specific individual(s)

Intracranial hematoma – blood collection within the substance of the brain

Jaundice – yellow to yellow-green skin discoloration

Joules – measurement of electric energy discharged by a defibrillator

Laryngoscope – instrument to visualize the vocal cords and assist in removing foreign bodies and insertion of endotracheal tube

Lobectomy – removal of a portion or segment of a lung

Magill forceps – angled forceps used to guide a tracheal tube into the windpipe or a nasogastric tube into the swallowing tube under direct vision; also used to remove foreign bodies in the throat

Meningitis – inflammation or infection of the linings of the brain and spinal cord

Molar pregnancy – abnormal form of pregnancy in which a non-viable fertilized egg implants and grows unrestrained as a mass

Mongolian spot – flat blue or gray birthmarks on a newborn or child most commonly located on lower back and buttocks; although they can look like bruises, they are normal and not a sign of child abuse or any other condition

Mononucleosis – usually caused by the Epstein-Barr virus (EBV); a general malaise followed by a set of signs and symptoms that may include high fever, severe sore throat, swelling of the lymph nodes, fatigue loss of appetite, muscle aches, enlargement of the spleen, swollen tonsils, and mild jaundice

Monospot (mono test) – used to help determine whether a person with symptoms has infectious mononucleosis (mono); frequently ordered along with a complete blood count (CBC) which determines whether the number of white blood cells (WBCs) is elevated and whether a significant number of reactive lymphocytes are present; if the mono test is initially negative the doctor may repeat the test one or more weeks later

Myoglobin – the special protein in muscle cells

N-acetylcystine – used in the management of (acetaminophen) overdose

Nasopharyngoscope – instrument to visualize the nose, pharynx and upper part of the larynx

Nephrology – the specialty for kidney disorders

Ophthalmology – the specialty for eyes

Orthopedic Surgery _ the specialty concerned with bony skeleton, joints and muscles [also – **Orthopods** and **Orthopedic service**]

Osmolar gap – the difference between measured and calculated osmolality in the serum of a blood sample

Otolaryngology – the specialty for Ear, Nose, Throat [also **Otorhinolaryngology**]

Packed cells – blood cells (usually red blood cells) with most of the fluid component removed

PACS – Picture Archiving and Communications System

Pediatrics – the specialty for disorders in children

Pancreatic amylase – digestive enzyme produced mainly by the pancreas

Pan-systolic – the entire time period spanning the first to the second heart sound

Pneumothorax – escape of air into the chest cavity from a puncture or break in the lung air sacks or tubes.

Pulmonary angiogram – x-ray assessment with dye injection to ascertain presence of pulmonary embolism or other vascular abnormality in the lungs

Pulmonary embolism – blood clot in lung vessel(s) formed in the venous side of circulatory system and breaking off to end up in the arteries of the lungs

QRS, QT Intervals – the measured time taken for the cardiogram tracing to traverse these specified predetermined points

Reduction and internal fixation – surgical operation to align broken bones and the use of internal screws, rods and bars to fix and maintain the alignment of the bone(s)

Rhabdomyolysis – a breakdown of muscle cells emptying their contents into the blood circulation and into the rigid envelope covering of the specific involved muscle(s)

Sclera – the opaque white lining sheath of the eyeball

Sub-Aortic Hypertrophic Cardiomyopathy – a genetic familial disorder where the left ventricular muscle mass